My Mental Health Matter: Beginnings

My Mental Health Matter: Beginnings

COACHING YOU THROUGH WELLNESS

Merisha Meisha

To order additional copies of this book, contact:
Xlibris
UK TFN: 0800 0148620 (Toll Free inside the UK)
UK Local: (02) 0369 56328 (+44 20 3695 6328 from outside the UK)
www.Xlibrispublishing.co.uk
Orders@Xlibrispublishing.co.uk
625890

Contents

The objectives of this book are

1. To share testimonies with people so that the benefit of salvation can be visible to all.
2. To use the testimonies shared to draw people closer to God so that their destiny can be defined in God who created them.
3. To reduce suicide rate through the sharing of testimonies with people, so that people can be filled with hope and be encouraged to live in hope for a better tomorrow.
4. To use the testimonies and experiences shared to increase people's faith so that fear is nullified and faith is amplified.
5. To use the testimonies to encourage people to keep the God Most High given vision alive so that depression can be depressed and Zoe enhanced.

Thank you, Lord, for taking me out from slavery into salvation and out from the well into wellness.

Quotations of the scriptures are taken from the King James Version of the Holy Bible except where stated otherwise.

This year, the year of the coronavirus pandemic, God is showing me that in a changing world, we need to look for new ways to praise Him. God is also showing me that He is too big for our brick houses and that we cannot contain Him in our boxes, which reminds me of a song titled the following:

'You are bigger than what people say. You are Jehovah.'

'I will speak of your testimonies bebore kings and
shall not be put to shame.'

— Psalms 119:46

'Never judge a book by its cover' – sounds cliché, but it's true.

In my weakest point, I'm at my strongest because God's grace locates
me with His power to prove His plan and purpose for me, and His plans
for my life must come to pass by His strengths.

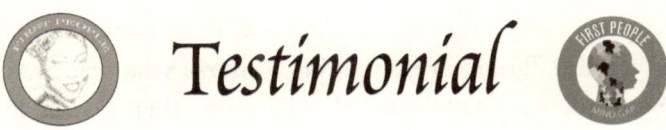

Testimonial

'To the law and testimony: if they speak not according to this word, it is because they have no light in them.'

— Isaiah 8:20 (King James Version)

———◆•◆•◆———

I, Irene Castellano, had a great opportunity to work with Merisha from 2019 to this day. She is a wonderful emotional coach who led me to be part of her beautiful project, First People Mind Gap, as a content editor.

I really appreciate having the opportunity to work with her, not just because of the amazing search for everyone's wellness but also because she is an exceptional professional in her work in the way that she is continually proactive in finding new ways to improve her work with modern technology and finding new creative ways to spread her message to get in touch with people's feelings.

Also, I have to emphasise on her incredible patience and understanding, which, in turn, make it much easier for me to manage my schedule effectively.

I'm really grateful. Thank you, Merisha.

<hr />

I first met Merisha when I was about to have life-saving surgery in September 2019.

Merisha was admitted in the same hospital as me and was staying in a hospital bed opposite mine. She could see that I was in a lot of pain and could barely stand up; she also noticed that there were no nurses coming to my aid. Therefore, she told the nurse who was attending to her to go and offer me help instead. The nurse then proceeded to my bedside and gave me more painkillers, which made me feel better and rest assured that I was being looked after.

Merisha prayed with and for me; she knew it was my first surgery, and she could see how frightened I was as I was going into surgery alone. Since leaving the hospital. Merisha has remained in contact with me, and she has really been that 'love and light' that I needed in someone at a traumatic time in my life.

I have also learned about Merisha's previous past traumatic health conditions, but in spite of her experiences, she has been creating an impact in her community by raising mental health awareness through the love of Christ to the people whom she meets in her daily journey. I have also heard how God is healing people through her ministry, First People Mind Gap, which is also raising mental health awareness, and People's People Mind Gap, which is a 'dance praise' to God for the destiny advancement of youths around the world.

I feel like Merisha has been doing extremely honourable work, particularly as she has begun to mentor me since 2020 during the

COVID-19 crisis after I informed her that I crave a closer relationship filled with revelations of Jesus Christ.

To top it all off, since our meeting, I have been gaining great insights on the mind of Christ through Merisha's mentoring, and I have found it easy to understand her methods of teaching.

I am extremely blessed to have met her, and I hope we can stay lifelong friends because I will never forget how Merisha assisted me in the hospital, not minding that she had a major operation in a matter of hours. It goes without saying that I am extremely grateful to God that He brought Merisha to me, for me, because of the immeasurable love that He has for me.

Ms Sarah E., West London

———————◆•◆•◆———————

I met Merisha in January 2019 at Winner Chapel Bible College; we were sitting beside each other. As time went on in class, we got to talking. It was then that I told her about my daughter's chest pain and my struggle as a single mother and living in a refuge. Merisha prayed for my daughter and also anointed her.

Merisha encouraged me with my own experience as a single mother and also kept in touch with me after we finished our Bible school.

I thank God for her and how she is always helping people because she assisted me with a lot of information and encouraged me to return to education.

I am happy I took her advice because I am now at the university, studying for my first degree in nursing. Also, Merisha prayed for my daughter's chest pain from 2019 until 2001. The chest pain that was so severe and lasted for years ceased after she prayed and anointed the chest, and now in 2021, my daughter's chest pain has never reoccurred to this day.

From my observations of Merisha's operations, I can see that she is really interested in the things about God, and she is deliberate at practicing them without being shy or afraid of who is laughing or watching her endeavours.

When I finally got my house, Merisha was the first person I confided in and invited immediately. Judging the timing of my life because of the events that had gone on, Merisha knew when to advise me to enrol for my degree, and I am now happy I made the decision to study nursing.

Returning to education in the year 2020 and attending my classes on Zoom has been the best thing that happened to me in the year of COVID-19 because it gives me the maximum amount of time to be flexible around my home and children.

I am very grateful to Merisha for supporting me with needed information and signposting me to places I have never heard of but that have aided my journey forward in life.

I am very thankful to God for matching my footpath with Merisha's because I truly believe that she is a destiny helper. She has impacted not just my life but those of my children too, and I bless the name of the Lord for my encounter with Merisha.

Ms Amina A, Grays, Essex

———◆———

I became born again in July 2016 at Winners Chapel Dartford. I took my BCC (basic certificate course) in February 2017. That is where I met a God-fearing woman whom I'm blessed to call my sister, Merisha.

Towards the end of the class, people were offering to drop people off at home or at the nearest stations to their homes if they were going in the same direction, and with God's intervention, Merisha lived not far from the station I needed to commute from. So at the end of the day, Merisha ensured that she reserved me a seat in her car and dropped me off at the station as well as picked up other students who were going towards her direction.

I went through many hardships, and without failing, anytime I needed Merisha, she was there selflessly. She would call to check up on me to make sure I was all right. She never judged me. She gave me Bible verses to read, and we would pray after our phone conversations. She also gave me advice on how to connect directly with God.

One thing I will always love about Merisha is her directness and bluntness, which is what I needed sometimes. She definitely is a God-fearing woman who has a big heart and a true soul, and I am blessed to have her in my life and call her my sister.

They say God brings people into your life at the time you need them, and I will always thank God again and again for his precious daughter Merisha because as well as God saving me, she did too.

I pray God continues to bless Merisha and gives her the wisdom and strength to carry out all she sets out to do while working for God as His ambassador on earth in the mighty name of Jesus Christ.

Ms Kiran L., South East London

———◆•◆•◆———

In the year 2006, I met Merisha in a medical centre back here in Sweden at a period when I was going though bereavement shortly after losing a baby via premature death.

I confided to Merisha about the news I and my family had just received at the time and told her that we were finding it difficult to deal with both what had just then happened and the preparation for the funeral.

Merisha offered a very good listening ear and offered to support us in any way she could. Although Merisha explained that she did not live in Sweden, I felt that I would like to keep in contact with Merisha because it felt good to see another woman in my local community willing to support me in my time of need.

Since then, Merisha kept in contact with me throughout her stay in Sweden. However, to my greatest surprise, before Merisha left Sweden during that period, she visited my home with flowers. This, for me, was a sign of her compassionate personality, which demonstrates a rare but genuine act of kindness from a stranger.

I have maintained a very close relationship with Merisha since knowing her because she is a person of great value and a good counsellor. Most importantly, since I knew Merisha, over the years, I have witnessed her grow steadily in her faith and in the work that she does in her community as an ambassador for Christ and an active mental health activist.

As well as this, Merisha is so passionate about the recovery and restoration of the health of people in that she takes steps to pray for people who are sick in the hospital.

In all, I noticed that Merisha is passionate about her work and a dedicated mental health activist who is not shy to announce her faith to anyone she encounters on how it has helped her to gain and maintain total wholeness in dealing with the affairs of her mental health wellness.

Mrs Nikechi Joseph, Sweden

 # Commemoration

This book has been written as a memorial to God for His wonderful acts in my life because He took me out from a suicidal place to a successful place.

This is in remembrance of the late John Stephen Ugo Ehikwe, who was born on 2 October in the United Kingdom and died by suicide on 17 June at New Cross Railway Station, London.

 # Acknowledgements

I thank God for your life. I thank you so much for obtaining your own copy of my book and for having the faith that you will gain strength from reading this book.

I thank God especially for making my life a testimonial so that I have plenty of testimonies to share with you. I thank God again for giving me the stamina to write this book, for staying with me throughout this book process, and for remaining with me throughout all other First People Mind Gap mental health projects.

I thank God for ordering my footsteps to the Living Faith Bible Church in October 2015. So I am sending a special thank-you to my spiritual father in faith, the bishop of the Living Faith Bible Church, also known as Winners Chapel International in Dartford, Kent.

I am sending out a massive thank-you to Dr AC, MD, for constantly encouraging me to stand firm with my faith as he too can see the massive turnaround in both my physical and mental health since I began to exercise and practice my faith in God's word and applying it to my life.

I am glad I took the courage and began to share my story with the people in my community who are suffering from anxiety, to help them see that there's a way out of a suppressed life caused by ill health and that they too can live a life of hope and light for the future.

I am thanking you, my friends and family members who emerged both from my mother's womb and from non-biblical parents, for believing in me.

I thank God for staying with me always; even when I did not know Him as my Lord, He was still with me, preparing the way for my refinement.

I thank my father for encouraging me to be the best of myself in everything that I do and for reassuring me of my potential and pointing out the values of education and self-discipline from childhood.

I thank my mother for joining hands with God to see that I arrived on earth safely and for being an overcomer of her own encounters in life and a very strong and beautiful woman with a heart-warming smile.

I thank God for the wonderful and beautiful life of Savannah DS. I am thanking Savannah also for her enthusiasm and encouragement throughout this book process and with all other First People Mind Gap mental health projects.

I thank God for my life tutors who saw potential in me and not dyslexia and for them really encouraging me to go for my goals in life because they believed in me and saw an able, courageous, and resilient woman rather than a disabled, stunted woman.

I really appreciate the productive team and other artists who have worked with me on this project to see its completion from its creation.

I did not write my book; all I did was type out the narratives into stories on pages. My life experience wrote out my book, which is formed by my walk of life, which means this book is not complete without the people who walked in and out of my life. So I thank you, everyone, for making those decisions that triggered our encounters and departures.

I would especially like to thank the following:

All those who took time out to be involved in the book conference for recoding and photography, I really appreciate you.

To all you people around the world who have been supportive and enthusiastic about My Mental Health Matter even when they did not know what it was all about, I say a massive thank-you for believing in the works that God has put in my hands.

Foreword

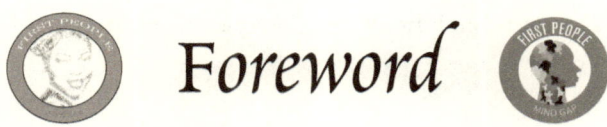

I am so honoured to be chosen from **_Sav-Santos-Beauty_** to comment on my experience of working on this book, _My Mental Health Matter: Beginnings_, because I am aware of Merisha's journey over the years and how she has used her weakness to become a strengthening hand for others to hold onto and climb higher in life.

Merisha has been providing both spiritual and mental health mentoring for both young people and adults in the United Kingdom as well as other parts in/and other continents, including Africa, Canada, and Sweden.

Merisha has survived many severe life-challenging experiences in her life. Amazingly, Merisha is now passing on her knowledge of how she survived these trials to the world for people to follow as a pathway to a successful breakthrough in life.

As a beautician and artist in the creative industry, I have worked closely with Merisha and benefitted from her versatile ways of performing and delivering her creative works.

I have observed her passionate ways during her mentoring sessions with me. I also noticed how important a role Merisha plays in her community for helping people who are not well guided but trying to find their way to a happier life to boost up their self-esteem, and in so doing, they are able to take control of their lives rather than take their lives in their own hands.

Her innovative and creative ways for supporting people via the mediums of poems and dancing are what make her work genuine and unique. Again, the way she is able to connect quickly with people makes her stand out in her area of work, especially when supporting individuals and families to gain back healthier lifestyles to maintain a better state of mind.

I am very proud to be associated with Merisha's projects, and I am happy to have dedicated my time into personally creating the logo for First People Mind Gap in support of the My Mental Health Matter programme that Merisha is dedicated to.

Ms Ruby JAS, Dos-Santostrindade

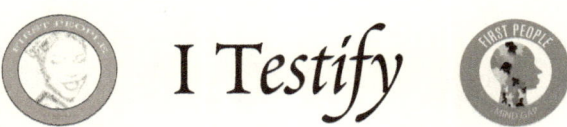

I Testify

No pupil graduates from a particular school and then goes to another school to participate in the graduation ceremony hosted especially for the students of that other school. With this result, I have returned as a Bible scholar from the Winners family to give all the glory to God almighty for blessing me with multiple testimonies and encounters which have truly turned my life from tumbling to testimonial.

I am also aware that if I am a sincere Bible student who is seeking the knowledge of God, to know the mind of God for me and mankind, then there is no graduation date from Bible school. This is because every reread of the scriptures reveals a fresh revelation to that scripture, which tells me that God is saying something new every day from something old. This is so that I can obtain the daily wisdom that I need each day and so forth to excel in faith with the day-to-day challenges that I may encounter.

I have begun my ministry of teaching youths the core disciplines of the ministry of Yeshua Hamashiach. I am still a registered student of Bible school because a good therapist must be supervised, and every good coach must be coached. As such, there should be dates of celebration for me to look forward to as dates of climbing up as a higher leader by qualifying to complete with joy multiple works that God puts in my hands for my ministry to grow and reach out to the right people.

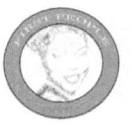 # God's Names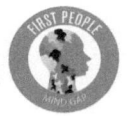

Learning to discover the meanings of this majestic God almighty helps me to begin to understand that the one and only living God is not a myth but a mysterious God whose mysteries turn into miracles. In addition, there is power in the name of God, but to experience the blessings in His name, one must be deeply conscious to plug into the meaningfulness of God's names before the encounters from confessing His names can be manifested. This is because God's names carry such weight that can deliver an instant testimony just by mentioning them – with the understanding of the essence and existence of the name mentioned while in warfare or during praise. When I call on the names of God while praising Him, I exalt His throne, and as I do so, He lifts me up and draws me nearer to Him. **Psalms 29:2 says, 'Give unto the Lord the glory due his name; worship the Lord in the beauty of holiness.'**

Whenever I call on the names of the LORD, I rest assured that He has heard me calling, and whenever I praise Him, I feel my joy renewed instantly because God does not want us to worry but rather bring our worries to Him. Praise is one of the ways that God mysteriously uses to quench the stubborn storms that are set to pull us down.

It is good to know the names of God because there are days when the devil will place an unexpected battle ahead of us; however, knowing God's names beforehand will be to our advantage.

We know God by calling His name in an appropriate manner, and we claim Him through the encounters we have from knowing Him. God's names help us identify Him by His mysteries and wonder – some, He called Himself, and others, the people of God called Him as they got to know Him by His works.

Authentic Names of God

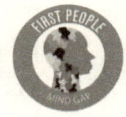

- Abir — He is the Mighty One of Jacob Isaiah 1:24).
- Adonai — He is the Lord (Genesis 15:2).
- Attiyq Youm — He is He that was before the Beginning of Time (Daniel 7:9, 13–14).
- Branch — He is the Branch (Zechariah 3:8).
- El Berith — He is the God of Israel, the Covenant-Keeping God (Judges 9:26).
- El Chuwl — He is the God Who Gave Birth (Psalms 139:13).
- El Deah — He is the God of Wisdom (1 Samuel 2:3).
- El Gibhor — He is the Mighty God (Isaiah 9:6).
- Eloah (Job 3:4 and 40:2)
- El Elyon — He is the Most High God (Genesis 14:18–20).
- El Olam — He is the Everlasting God (Isaiah 40:28–31).
- Elohim — He is the Strong Creative God of Power and Might (Genesis 1:1; 1 Kings 8:23; Isaiah 40:2; Jeremiah 33:1).
- El Roi — He is the God Who Sees and Opens our Eyes (Genesis 16:13).

- El Shaddia — He is the Lord God Almighty and the All-Sufficient God (Genesis 17:1; Micah 2:1).
- Eyaluth — He is Strength (Psalms 22:19).
- Goal — He is the Redeemer (Job 19:55).
- Jehovah — Yahweh is the covenant name of God. Likewise, He is the Self Existence – 'I AM Who I Am and Will Be Who I Say I Am because I Am Life' (Exodus 3:8).
- Jehovah Raah — He is a caring Shepherd (Psalms 23:1).
- Jehovah Jireh — He is the Lord who Provides and Foresees the Future (Genesis 22:14).
- Jehovah M' Kaddesh — He is the Lord who sanctifies one to make whole and sets aside to make holy (Leviticus 20:7–8).
- Jehovah Nissi — He is the Lord Our Banner, a victorious God Who lifts us up in Victory (Exodus 17:15; Psalms 4:6).
- Jehovah Prohe — He is the Lord Who Heals (Jeremiah 30:17 and 3:22; Isaiah 61:1; Exodus 15:22–26).
- Jehovah Shalom — He is the Lord of Peace and Perfection Who takes care of our Welfare (Judges 6:24).
- Jehovah Tsidkenu — He is the Lord of Justice and Righteousness (Jeremiah 23:6).
- Jehovah Rohi — He is the Lord Our Shepherd (Psalms 23).
- Jehovah Shammah — He is the Lord who is always present (Ezekiel 48:35).
- Jehovah Sabaoth — He is the commander and the Lord of hosts (Isaiah 1:24).
- Kanna — He is a Jealous God (Exodus 20:5; Isaiah 9:7).
- Kadosh — He is the Holy One of Israel (Isaiah 40:25).
- Magan — He is the Shield (Psalms 18:30).
- Palet — He is the Deliverer (Psalms 18:2).
- Qanna — He is a Jealous God (Exodus 20:5).
- Shaphat — He is the God, the Judge (Genesis 18:25).
- Stone — He is solid as stone yet an unbreakable God (Genesis 49:24).
- Soter — He is the Saviour (Luke 1:4, 7).
- Tsaddiq — He is the Righteous One (Psalms 7:9).
- Tsur — He is God, Our Rock (Isaiah 30:29).

- Yahweh — He is the Lord Jehovah (Deuteronomy 6:4).
- Yahweh Ghmolah — He is the God of Recompense (Jeremiah 51:6).
- Yahweh Maccaddeshem — He is the God who Sanctifies (Exodus 21:13; Leviticus 20:8).
- Yahweh Rapha — He is the God Who Heals (Exodus 15:26).
- Yeshua — He is the Saviour who would Save (Isaiah 43:3; Mark 12 [Jewish Bible]).
- Yomin — He is the Ancient of Days (Daniel 7:22 [Jewish Bible]).

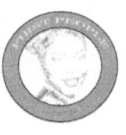

Other Bona Fide Names of God

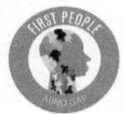

- Advocate (1 John 2:1)
- Almighty God (Revelation 1:8)
- Alpha as seen in (Revelation 1:8)
- Alpha and Omega (Revelation 22:13)
- Amen (Revelation 3:14)
- Angel of the Lord (Genesis 16:17)
- Anchor (Hebrews 6:19)
- Anointed One (Psalms 2:2)
- Anchor (Hebrews 6:19)
- Apostle (Hebrews 3:14)
- Author and Finisher of our Faith (Hebrews 12:2)
- Beginning (Revelation 21:6)
- Beloved (Ephesians 1:6)
- Bishop of Souls (1 Peter 5:4)
- Branch (Isaiah 11:1)
- Bread of Life (John 6:35)
- Bridegroom (Matthew 9:15)

- Bright and Morning Star (Revelation 22:16)
- Carpenter (Mark 6:13)
- Chief Cornerstone (Ephesians 2:20)
- Chief Shepherd (1 Peter 5:4)
- Christ (Matthew 1:16)
- Comforter (Jeremiah 8:18)
- Consolation of Israel (Luke 2:25)
- Dayspring (Luke 1:78)
- Day Star (2 Peter 1:19)
- Deliverer (Romans 11:26)
- Desire of Nations (Haggai 2:7)
- Door (John 10:9)
- Despots [He is the Lord] (Acts 4:2)
- Emmanuel (Matthew 1:23)
- End (Revelation 21:6)
- Everlasting Father (Isaiah 9:6)
- Faithful and True Witness (Revelation 3:14)
- Father (Isaiah 63:16)
- First Fruits (1 Corinthians 15:23)
- First and Last (Revelation 1:17)
- Foundation (Isaiah 28:16)
- Fountain (Zechariah 13:1)
- Friend of Sinners (Matthew 11:19)
- Gate for the Sheep (John 10:7)
- Gift of God (2 Corinthians 9:15)
- God (John 1:1)
- Glory of God (Isaiah 41:14)
- Good Shepherd (John 10:11)
- Governor (Matthew 2:6)
- Great Shepherd (Hebrews 13:20)
- Guide (Psalms 48:14)
- Head of the Church (Ephesians 5:23; Colossians 1:18)
- High Priest (Hebrews 6:20 and 3:1)
- Holy One (Mark 1:24)
- Holy One of Israel (Isaiah 41:14)
- Horn of Salvation (Luke 1:69)

- Hypsistos [He is the highest] (Matthew 21:9)
- I Am (Exodus 3:14)
- Image of the Invisible God (Colossians 1:15)
- Immanuel (Matthew 1:23)
- Jehovah (Psalms 83:18)
- Jesus (Matthew 1:21)
- Judge (Acts 10:42; Psalms 7:8 and 96:13)
- King of Israel (Matthew 27:42)
- King of Jews (Mark 15:26)
- King of Kings (1 Timothy 6:15; Revelation 19:16)
- Lamb of God (John 1:29)
- Last Adam (1 Corinthians 15:45)
- Life (John 11:25)
- Light of the World (John 8:12)
- Lion of the Tribe of Judah (Revelation 5:5)
- Living Water (John 4:10)
- Lord of Lords (1 Timothy 6:15)
- Man of Sorrows (Isaiah 53:3)
- Master (Matthew 8:19 and 26:18)
- Mediator (1 Timothy 2:5)
- Melekh [He is King] (Isaiah 5:1, 5, and 41:21)
- Messiah (John 1:41; Daniel 9:25)
- Mighty God (Isaiah 9:6)
- Morning Star (Revelation 22:16)
- Nazarene (Matthew 2:23)
- Omega (Revelation 1:8)
- Only Begotten Son (John 3:16)
- Passover Lamb (1 Corinthians 5:7)
- Physician (Matthew 9:12)
- Potentate (1 Timothy 6:15)
- Priest (Hebrews 4:15)
- Prince of Peace (Isaiah 9:6)
- Prophet (Acts 3:22; Matthew 21:11)
- Propitiation (1 John 1:49)
- Purifier (Malachi 3:3)
- Rabbi (1:49)

- Ransom (1 Timothy 2:6)
- Redeemer (Job 19:25; Isaiah 41:14)
- Refiner (Malachi 3:2)
- Refuge (Isaiah 25:4)
- Resurrection and Life (John 11:25)
- Righteousness (Jeremiah 23:26)
- Rock (1 Corinthians 10:4; Deuteronomy 32:4)
- Root of David (Revelation 5:5)
- Rose of Sharon (Songs of Solomon 2:1)
- Ruler of God's Creation (Revelation 3:14)
- Sacrifice (Ephesians 5:2)
- Saviour (2 Samuel 22:47; Luke 1:47; John 4:42)
- Seed of David (2 Timothy 2:8)
- Seed of Woman (Genesis 3:15)
- Second Adam (1 Corinthians 15:47)
- Servant (Isaiah 42:1; Matthew 12:18)
- Shepherd and Bishop of Souls (1 Peter 2:25; Psalms 79:13 and 95:7)
- Shiloh (Genesis 49:10)
- Son of God (Luke 1:35; Mark 1:1)
- Son of Man (Matthew 18:11 and 20:28)
- Son of Mary (Mark 6:3)
- Son of the Most High (Luke 1:32)
- Stone (Isaiah 28:16)
- Sun of Righteousness (Malachi 4:2)
- Teacher (John 3:2)
- Theotes the Godhead (Romans 1:20)
- True Vine (John 15:1)
- Truth (John 14:6)
- Vine (John 15:1)
- Way, Truth, and Life (John 1:1)
- Wonderful Counsellor (Isaiah 9:6).
- Word (John 1:1)
- Yahweh (Psalms 135:2)

 Salvation

There are seven rules that govern our prayer life until the perfect day of our union with God, but we are to reconcile first with God before we reconnect.

'Ye are of God, little children, and have overcome them: because greater is he that is in you than he that is in the world.'

— 1 John 4:4 (KJV)

Having an awareness of the existence of God is the starting point of acknowledging that God is the creator of the universe. Then receiving God as your Lord and heavenly Father through the help of the Holy Spirit secures your salvation and protects you against sinful nature if you take conscious steps to walk on the desired path under the law that God has chosen for us in the **Ten Commandments**, which are written in Exodus 20.

Accepting the salvation of God over your life is admitting that you are coming into a covenant to serve God through the help of His Holy Spirit; this is a commitment of your **love** for God. Meanwhile, you demonstrate this love for God through loving the things of God and by loving your neighbour as yourself.

These are the two greatest commandments that would guide you to the heart of God, but I would like to encourage you to give your life to God if you have not yet already done so. Otherwise, if you would like to re-dedicate your life to God, it would be better to do so now before venturing into the chapters of this book so that your experience in encountering light from reading this book will be validated by heaven.

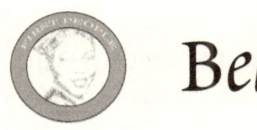 # Believers

'Behold, what manner of love the Father hath bestowed upon us that we should be called the sons of God: therefore, the word knoweth us not because it knew him not.'

— 1 John 3:1

The spotlight is on believers as non-believers are closely watching the behaviour of those who believe before they too can come about believing because they judge by what they see believers do as what believers believe in and not by what they hear believers say they believe **(1 Thessalonians 2:8–16)**.

Why believers need to believe is because the works of the Father are on believers so that non-believers can see the works of the Father in the life of a believer.

A woman saw me singing praises on the street one Sunday afternoon.

She said, 'Why are you so happy and I'm so sad?'

I stopped singing and went to speak with her because my ministry is all about putting smiles on the faces of people and telling them that they are loved and special. Also, God wants for them, more than anything else, to be well in both their bodies and their minds.

At the end of our conversation, she admitted that she was confused about the way 'Christianity' works because of the attitudes of some Christians who keep clapping in the church buildings yet don't share the joy in the community.

A part of the reason why you hear people not coming to the calling of the gospel and why some people stop believing in God is that they are not seeing the hospitality sessions among the brethren who claim they believe and act in love. It is also common to see certain persons depart from the building of the church because the fellowshipping aspect of that gathering has left the building **(Hebrews 13:16)**. We are encouraged not to neglect doing good and sharing it with one another, for this is what will please God. In other words, there are gatherings that God will frown upon if not done. This manner of fellowship may fall into a selfish and sinful manner of coordinating, and we know this through the expression of God's words and His distance from our means.

 What About Sin?

Sin is when we disobey God, but God is always giving us fresh opportunities to drop our old ways and pick up the new ways for our renewal of faith.

Sin stains one's life and makes them stink before it sinks them. When sin sticks out more in a person's life, that person will not just sink but also stink spiritually, especially if that person has recently had a close walk with God but recently withdrawn. When the sin in a person increases, the God in them decreases **(1 John 3)**.

Hold on to this and know that the LORD is not slack:

**'Behold, the Lord's hand is not shortened
that it cannot save; neither his ear heavy
that it cannot hear. But your iniquities have
separated between you and your God, and
your sins have hid his face from you, that he
[will] not hear.'**

— Isaiah 59:1–2

Sin keeps us far from God in a way that we do not receive revelation from Him, therefore leading to our communication being cut off from Him.

My dear friend, kindly accept this simple prayer of salvation in your heart and allow God's Spirit to dwell in your spirit as one.

My Lord Yeshua,

I thank you for dying on the cross to take away my sins. I am sorry my ways haven't been according to your commandments. I ask you to please come into my heart and cleanse it of all wrongdoings. I now accept you as my Saviour and Lord and promise not to return to the ways of the world. So help me God.

> **'And the Spirit of the LORD will rest upon him, the spirit of wisdom and understanding, and the spirit of counsel and might, the spirit of knowledge and of the fear of the LORD.'**
>
> **— Isaiah 11:2**

Refer to **Matthew 6:33**. Say that when we seek God's kingdom and its righteousness, first, every other thing that men are dying for would be added unto us. Remember that God will not add unto you what is killing other men or holding them away from the word and pulling them more into the world. Rather, He knows what you need that is good for you. So according to His will for you, He will add to you what will increase and elevate you as you obey in the mighty name of *Yeshua Hamashiach.*

Be blessed as you read on. I pray that light bursts forth and God gives you both wisdom and understanding to hear what His Spirit is saying to you and that the name of the Lord will be praised and glorified.

Amen.

Chapter I

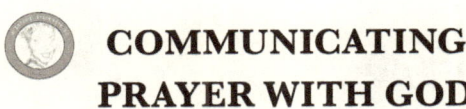

COMMUNICATING PRAYER WITH GOD

 Prayer

It is important that we keep the prayer altar burning, for we know not when the enemy would sneak in at night like a thief to afflict us as we resettle not against flesh and blood but against principalities, against powers, against the rulers of the darkness of this world, against spiritual wickedness in high places. Therefore, take unto you the whole armour of God that ye may be able to withstand the evil day and, having done all, to stand **(Ephesians 6:12, paraphrased)**.

> **'Praying always with all prayer and supplication in the Spirit and watching thereunto with all perseverance and supplication for all saints.'**
>
> **— Ephesians 6:18**

Prayer is one of the ways God uses to communicate with us so that we can obtain things of the Spirit from Him. We take cover under the shadow of God when we stay connected to God in prayer because the devil is always busy looking for which one of the saints to pull down. If we don't obtain wisdom from God through prayers, the devil would succeed in seeing that we do not become successful with the work that our heavenly Father has given us to do.

We obtain mercy and favour from God during prayer time, so it is important to pen prayers asking for mercy so that our prayers can be heard and so that we can be delivered from any known and unknown satanic oppression that is forbidding our progress. Praying also helps to build up our faith so that we can come boldly before God to remind Him of His promises.

◯ Praying Times ◉

Praying at all times in these times, in the days that we are in now, is very crucial. This is mostly to maintain a healthy prayer lifestyle so that we can cancel devilish dreams and demonic attacks with the prayers that we render to the Most High God. These are the words that we declare while praying regardless of our busy lifestyles or what others assume of our praying habits (praying without ceasing). This remains the key to winning without failing, which brings us nearer to the Most High without ending.

However, some may wander off; surely, there should be appropriate times assigned to pray accurately in our home surroundings, in our work environment, and even in the public space so that we are not seen as a nuisance or concern to others.

It is true that when a person is radical with their prayer, they can be perceived as if something is not OK with their mental health by those who do not understand fully that prayers should be declared boldly. However, there is a place and time when this should be done. Just like the fact that we cannot just stop and eat any type of food anywhere just because we are hungry, one should have the discipline to coordinate what they say in prayer, where and when they say it and to the hearing of who, and be deliberate with this action. This is because as many as there are angels doing good deeds, so are there millions of demons that have attached themselves to things on this planet to demolish the good works of men and deform their character to conform to evil.

> **'Rejoice evermore. Pray without casing in everything. Give thanks.'**
>
> **— 1 Thessalonians 5:16–18**

Bearing this in mind, there are other acceptable and discreet ways to remain in prayer always. However, this does not mean exercising prayer for twenty-four hours a day without giving the mind/brain a break to process other things in one's life or to enjoy the beauty of peace without a noisy and constantly busy mind.

◯ Creative Prayer Times and Methods ⊛

Knowing now that there is a time and place for prayer, what is the time and place for prayer?

There are no specific times to pray, just like there are no specific set times for all to eat as person to person hungers at different times in the course of the day. Nevertheless, there are secluded times set aside in the day as the best mealtimes. This is relevantly the same for prayer times, but it is up to the individual to align their spirit with the Spirit of the Most High on what time would be best set as a meeting time for prayer. The meeting point can also be concluded by the person after this agreement is acknowledged by the Most High.

This does not mean that you cannot pray outdoors as you can also apply being discreet. Then you pray outdoors by coining into your heart and staying heartily connected in your prayers. Some of the methods are via praying in your mind; the same way that there is a lot of communication between the head and the mind, prayers can also form patterns through this channel but to the Most High God.

Apart from the obvious method of praying in the mind, there are other ways you can pray discreetly without bringing any outside attention to yourself because prayers are enforced by bold declarations. These include using headphones pinned to your garments from the inside without necessarily having the phone on you or switching off your phone to avoid interference from message alerts or incoming calls. In addition to this, a mask can also be worn to make the movement of the lips less obvious in the absence of headphones, or it can be used in conjunction with the headphones.

Entering His Presence

Prayer is the key to life and the real food for life, but we need to know how to come into the presence of the Most High at the time of prayer. When you call God into your presence, you will enjoy His presence. How we enter the presence of Jehovah or God is important. Thus, **Psalms 100:4** tells us this: **'Enter His gate with thanksgiving and into His courts with praise: be thankful unto Him and bless His name.'** Entering with thanksgiving and praise, however, would mean that we would need to come with our hearts, delightful to receive from the Lord in spite of our challenges, exactly as it is spoken in **Proverbs 23:26**: **'My son, give me thine heart, and let thine eyes observe my ways.'**

Will you go for a job interview without preparation or dressing appropriately? Will you visit the queen if invited without knowing what the protocol of your visitation to the palace is?

We will not go to a king without fully being prepared – what more entering into the presence of the King of Kings in a dishonouring way? So if our answer to these questions is no, why then should we casually walk into the presence of the Most High carelessly without observing the ways that He wants us to meet with Him? Unlike when preparing to meet a man, where the focus is based on bodily appearance and the person is judged by their materialistic content, when preparing to meet with the King of Kings, the contents of our heart are what God is looking at to weigh our motives. This is like the case of King Amaziah, who did what was right in the sight of the LORD but not with a loyal heart; God knew this, and his service was not accepted in the end **(2 Chronicles 25:2)**.

Entering the presence of the Lord does not require any silver or gold coins from our pockets. Rather, we come as we are with our hearts and prepare to receive the purification of the Lord so our minds are reset, leaving us confident to deal boldly with those challenges that we came to present to the Lord. His word says, **'Come unto me, all ye that labour and are heavy laden, and I will give you rest' (Matthew 11:28)**.

There are too many things interfering with our relationship with God, from the government's new rules, implementing reinforcement at the place of work, and the re-enactment of poor practices copied from our peers to social media distractions that hold us bound. These are some examples among many things that can remove the appearance of the Holy Spirit from us when we come to seek the face of God.

Some of the good practices before we enter the presence of God – even if it is in our homes, at our place of work, or even when we are in the midst of a crowd – include learning how to switch off the external noise internally and mentally capturing a space of silence in our minds. By doing this, we are creating room for the Holy Spirit to occupy that part of our psyche. Learning these skills is important because when the enemy comes, he comes without warning, and one of the most powerful defence tools of a believer is keeping still yet turning on the fire with prayers.

Remember – when practicing this, you cannot expect to shut the world up because you want to pray. So adopt an attitude of going back into yourself to trigger a response from the one who resides in you. Although learning this vital skill needs heart-to-heart engagement with God as God is a hearty supernatural being, you need to look up to Him to send the wisdom for you to activate this.

We ought to pray without ceasing and be mindful so as not to allow our gadgets to stop the moment the answer to our prayer comes to us. This includes picking up the phone the moment the Holy Ghost is about to deposit inspiration or instruction to us; this could be the same moment that that testimony is stolen or delayed by the enemy, who is always working against God's plan in the life of the people. The caller could be a genuine caller on the other end, but the enemy's ways to rob us of the presence of the LORD are plenty. So we must pray to remain sensitive and ask the Holy Spirit for the spirit of discernment so that we can judge a certain pattern.

I have a saying: 'My phone is made for me. I am not made for my phone.' Therefore, when it rings of its own accord, without my official agreement to engage with it, it will take my accord to pick up the call or call the caller back at a time suitable for me because it rang at a time that suits it without my consent, so I am not obliged to engage in it.

How would you feel if I turned up late to your after receiving an invitation on more than one occasion and did not seem bothered? What if I picked up every call that had come through my phone and replied to every single text message before acknowledging your presence?

If this happened to me over time, I would feel as though you didn't appreciate my friendship and, most importantly, you did not value my time, and I would have to rethink how much of my time I put on the table for you. Think about it. This is how much of God's time we waste forgetting that God has given us our freedom, but He has our time, and we will give Him an account of how we have spent our time at the end of time. Also, not spending quality time with God when we come to His presence is dismissing the knowledge that He is a jealous God **(Exodus 20:5)**.

What are you ready to turn away for God so that you can hear from Him?

It is our obedience that would help God deliver our request speedily into our hands. For example, when Moses was approaching the burning bush in **Exodus 3:5**, the LORD spoke to Moses again, telling him not to come nearer until he took off his shoes, for he was entering a holy ground. Moses did as he was told, and then he was able to receive the mandate and instructions for the Ten Commandments that God had prepared for him to take back to the people.

◐ Merciful Father ◉

'For [it] is of the Lord's mercies that we are not consumed because His compassions fail not.'

— Lamentations 3:22–23

We ought to thank God for His mercy, which has preserved and protected our lives so far, before asking Him for His grace to uphold our being. Asking for mercy is the first prayer we should say when we come into the presence of the Lord. By asking for mercy first, we are getting our hearts ready to flee from guilt before laying our requests to Him. Asking for mercy first before laying down any petitions in front of the Lord shows God that although we are aware that we are sinners, we are not proud of the sin itself, but rather, we want to repent from sin and draw nearer to God.

Therefore, so as not to hinder our prayers, we should first acknowledge our wrongdoing and then come clean before the Lord with clear minds and bodies that are full of light to receive the Holy Spirit and transfer it to our bodies and, in so doing, hear what the Holy Spirit is about to communicate to our spirit. Bear in mind that we too need to be merciful to others; otherwise, we are not qualified to request that mercy prevail our offences, known or unknown.

'If we say that we have not sinned, we deceive ourselves, and the truth is not in us.'

— 1 John 1:8

'Wherefore God resisteth the proud but giveth grace unto the humble.'

—James 4:6

'Be ye merciful, as your Father also is merciful; forgive, and ye shall be forgiven.'

— Luke 6:36–37 (paraphrased)

Confession Prayer

God is quick to forgive us; however, He wants us to confess our sins, both known and unknown.

So What Is Our Bit to Do?

God is a convent-keeping God, and He is always available to play His part as He has already committed to it in His word. In like manner, it is our responsibility to confess our sins, and when we do, we feel lighter in our spirit, as if we have dropped a load of satanic language off our lives.

Proverbs 28:13 says that when we confess our sins, we would prosper, but when we hide them, we will not prosper or obtain mercy. As we need mercy to obtain grace from God so that we can both be fervent and prevail in prayer, it is wise to confess for us our sins before engaging in prayer so that our prayers are not hindered **(1 John 1:9)**.

◐ **Giving Thanks to the Father** ⊛

**'In everything, give thanks: for this is the will
of God concerning you.'**

— 1 Thessalonians 5:18

We should give God thanks in advance for answering our prayers even before we have prayed to Him, knowing with an assurance that He has heard us. This is the kind of faith God wants us to demonstrate to show that we are assured and trust in Him and that we reassure Him as believers.

See the example that the Messiah showed us when He gave thanks to God before performing these miracles. The Messiah was called to the grave where Lazarus lay dead after four days; however, the first thing He did after rolling away the stone from the grave was give thanks to the Father. Again, at Galilee, when the Messiah performed the miracle of feeding the five thousand with five loaves of bread and two fishes, the first thing that He did before breaking the bread was give thanks to the Father **(John 11:41–42)**.

According to **John 6:11**, when you can see every reason to be thankful, you will have a good reason to be joyful as joy and thanksgiving go hand in hand. The more you give thanks, the more the oil of gladness is perfumed into your life, activating the spirit of joy in your life for you to keep rejoicing.

We thank God in anticipation for the answers to our prayers even before we have seen the results of our prayers. The expression for our joy before God triggers His presence in our midst during and after our prayers, and He multiplies whatever we came to give Him thanks for in surplus.

For example, when we thank God for revelations, there would be an outpouring of testimonies as a result of our thanksgiving.

Praying with joy does not absolve sorrow from our hearts, but it can exempt us from the sorrowful situation and release our minds from pain. I cannot emphasise enough how deadly it is to let go of one's joy, especially on a road that looks like a dead end. As a matter of truth, whenever you approach such a junction in life, it is time to retain your joy the most because the enemy knows that to empty everything from the person, first, it needs to steal their joy so that it can leave them dry. This is why Isaiah said that it is with joy we can obtain anything from the Lord **(Isaiah 12:3)**.

With broken hearts, we are not able to receive anything. This is why one of the enemies' tools to steal our joy is by bringing frightful challenges into our lives so that we can remain in fear and be absent of joy **(Proverbs 17:22)**.

Challenges come to us like a ton of bricks. Yes, this is true, and although it seems as if our world is collapsing in front of us (and other times, it may look as if there is nothing to live for or look forward to in life), the word of God is telling us to rejoice evermore **(1 Thessalonians 5:16)**.

It is when we choose to remain in joy that our joy will be topped up, and then we are liberated to the topmost. How?

Remember the testimonies that the LORD your God has given to you. Recall them and dance round with joy. Then take them as a point of reference to Jehovah; present them in your singing while exulting His name. Demonstrate that He is mighty to deliver you again this time as He did the last time, all by Himself, because He is a faithful God.

The moment you activate your thanksgiving mood, your joy is re-enacted because you cannot be thankful and not joyful, as Bishop Oyedepo puts it, and you cannot be joyful without being able to think of anything to be thankful for.

When you give thanks to God, you are showing your gratitude towards Him. However, if the situation is seemingly terrible and you cannot think of any immediate testimonies or apparent reasons to be grateful for, think of the breath you breathe daily for free. Make that be a good enough reason to give thanks to the one who created you and sustained you by His breath each day, from dawn to dusk. So remain encouraged, and when life seems dark because the light has been stolen from you, do not moan with your last drop of breath. Rather, be engaged with the psalms that say to let everything that has breath praise the LORD (**Psalms 150:6**). As a reminder to those Israelites who complained about their escape from Egypt, the Bible records that the people were destroyed by the Destroyer (**1 Corinthians 10:10**).

Time with the Father

Time alone with God is awesome, so be dedicated and deliberate in delegating a set time aside with the LORD because the Holy Spirit is intentional with us. Setting time aside for God to welcome His presence does not have to be an awkward task because God will work with our time as long as we keep to His set time.

Remember that God has given you your freedom, but He has our time, so He will never arrange a time with you that will jeopardise your official work schedule. However, if your work schedule infringes with the time He wants to spend with you and your heart is willing to go with His leading, He can make your work plans work best for you by moving things around at your workplace so that you are given a new schedule altogether which will enable you to stay in His peaceful presence when you are called into it. Another aspect is that when God sees in your heart that you are desperate to stay under His wings, the Holy Spirit can bless you with a better job that has more financial benefits and less working hours, including having the Sabbath Day off as part of your days off work.

Different times work for different people; likewise, the Holy Ghost will call you into His presence at a time that it knows will draw you closer to Him so that you are able to fulfil God's planned purpose for your life. For example, the Holy Ghost can begin to wake you up constantly at a set hour in the early hours of the morning; be sensitive to pick this up in your spirit and allow the Spirit of God to work in you, and be mindful not to mistake this time as toilet time. However, when in doubt, work on it, and God will work with you because God is the author of peace and not of confusion. So He will never bring you anything that distresses you. It may be inconvenient for you, but it will not be to distress you; rather, it will bless you **(1 Corinthians 14:33)**.

In the world, they say 'the early bird eats the worm'. In the word of God, those who seek God early shall find Him, and He will give them His wisdom and riches. When you wake up early and you present yourself in the sight of the LORD, you are honouring Him with your time. In return, He will give you His wisdom that He has not released to anyone yet, but it is up to you to follow the lead of His instructions, which will grant you the riches that the LORD talks about in **Proverbs 8:17**.

In 2017, I attended the world bible school lectured by Pastor David Oyedepo of the Winners Chapel headquarters in Nigeria. I heard him sharing one of his testimonies of how he had once told God to make his three hours of sleep as solid as eight hours of restful sleep at night. I kept this testimony in my mind and later on used it in December of that same year during **Shiloh**. Shiloh occurs yearly at the Winners family in a period set aside so that the members can infuse themselves with the presence of the LORD.

After my return from Shiloh that same year, I will never forget the reception I received from people from different walks of life because of the questions I was asked, such as 'What was your holiday location?' I remember having a business meeting with an official agent from the Greenwich council in Charlton House, London. This gentleman could not get over the fact that I was glowing so much and had not left UK soil. In his own words, 'God is really real'.

That was Mr. Greenford's first time meeting me in his life, yet because of the glow I was wearing, he thought I had been on holiday for weeks and had just gotten back in time for the meeting. The holy truth is that I was simply basking in the glory of the King, the almighty God, as a result of presenting myself in His presence on the Shiloh grounds for five days at Living Faith International in Dartford, Kent. The King of Kings poured on me blessings that I could not touch but could feel and that could be seen by everyone else as its effect was that powerful – that powerful that only God can do.

What Is Shiloh?

A lot of people have asked me the question 'What is Shiloh?' whenever I say I am getting ready for Shiloh. Shiloh is a season of God gathering the people together to release their overdue blessings to them. The following verses and chapters make mentions of Shiloh for you to review:

- **Joshua 18 — 'The whole congregation of the children of Israel came together for to hear from the Lord at Shiloh.'**
- **1 Samuel — 'When Hannah came back from Shiloh, she made love with her husband [who was] named Elkanah and became pregnant. This pregnancy [led] to the birth of Samuel.'**
- **1 Samuel 3:21 — 'And the LORD appeared again in Shiloh: for the LORD revealed himself to Samuel in Shiloh by the word of the LORD.'**

When God calls the people together, He appears to the people, and when He is in the midst of the people, He does not leave them the same way He met them but blesses them.

◯ **Time to Pray** ⊛

Dedicating time for God is paramount for our prayer life because in God's kingdom, nothing is a coincidence, so nothing should happen randomly as God is a God of time and order.

In the course of our busyness, we go on about how our business is too busy for us to mind the business of our Father, sometimes even in that ministry that God Himself has delivered to us to mind for Him. However, we seem to forget about Him in the day's business and are too busy with things that do not have anything to do with taking a moment aside to appreciate that the one who sent us is still with us.

Steal a minute for your creator in the corner of your work store or creative workshop and say, *'Father, I thank you, LORD'* a few good times. Notice if you don't feel refreshed and relieved of any issues that may have been hanging around you. You may even receive instant inspiration on how to resolve that matter, if any.

Initially, at the beginning of the year 2020, when I decided to take my writing projects seriously, I began to get panic attacks from the enemy of progress (the devil). I recognised the symptoms but could not do anything to stop them from happening, even if I read books on anxiety, some from the spiritual point of view based on the word of God and others written from a psychological point of view.

Yes, I got a lot of enrichment from these books and began putting some suggestions into my daily practices, yet the phobia that I would not be able to complete my writing project did not leave me until I began to give God thanks for enabling me to write. I sat right in front of a blank screen and gave thanks even though my head was full of a hundred books to write. I was injected with fear, so I could not pen my point to print.

I will never forget the morning of 20 April 2020. Immediately after giving God thanks in my study ark, I heard the Holy Spirit speak straight to my own spirit, and what was said to me still stays with me to this day as I heard, *'Stay with me. I am with you always. Don't be afraid to do whatever I ask you to do.'*

Dear friends, I could not touch on what emotions I had felt when I heard this, but to say I did not know how to react would be an understatement. I did not know if I should cry, sing, dance on top of the table, or even hide under the table. However, the one thing that stood out for sure was that I was filled with joy for receiving direct comfort from the heavens above. This gave me such a boost of energy that I spent more time thanking God even in the midst of my activities. To the glory of God, today I have a few of my completed creative projects that I am benefitting from, and now I am able to share them with you and the rest of the world.

Another thing about our willingness to create time for God is that when we do, He will make it His duty to create time for us in the daytime, which allows us to be with Him. For example, the Holy Spirit can wake anyone up at a set time early in the morning without the aid of an alarm, and this would be the order of the day for us so that we can gain extra time during the day to enable quality time with Him.

I testify that the following blessing is a venture of wishful thinking. I watched a woman of God share her testimony on YouTube, hearing about how the Holy Ghost wakes her up so early in the morning to enable her pray at a certain time within the holy hours when spiritual warfare is taking place. I could not believe my amazement when, that very same night, I went to bed, and at that same hour she had mentioned in her video, I was woken up by the angels that only the Holy Spirit of God could have arranged on my behalf on the morning of 6 December 2020. As proof that this is not a coincidence, these angels keep tweeting at this set time and waking me up.

I am indeed grateful to God because He is giving me ample time to stay with Him as well as complete a few tasks before I begin my set work for the day.

◐ Word Sword ◉

You are what you eat. The scriptures that you swallow on the days that you are sober are the scriptures that would jump out from your mouth on the days that you are feeling sick. To stop that sickness, you will need to retrieve the word you have in you. Even if the situation proves to be stubborn, with your constant resistance to firing the word of God at that ankle of challenge, you are bound to win that battle and overcome the obstacle.

The word of God is my anti-sickness tablet; it is quick and powerful and sharper than any two-edged sword **(Hebrews 4:12)** in that it pierces through the soul and spirit and the joints and bone marrow.

The word of God is real because of His spoken and written word. I personally could not put it better than this apart from adding that my invisible God is so real in my life because of His visible encounters with me. So I use myself when someone asks me how I know God is real.

I say, 'In His word.'

Saying this does not convince most people, who proceed with more inquisitive questions, which makes me tell them to take a look at me and see the reality of God in me.

I say, 'Take a look at me because . . . I am living proof of Hebrews 4:12 and many other words that have been altered out of the mouth of God.'

'For as the rain cometh down and the snow from heaven and returneth not thither but watereth the earth and maketh it bring forth and bud that it may give seed to the sower and bread to the eater, so shall my word be that goeth forth out of my mouth: it shall not return unto me void, but it shall accomplish that which I please, and it shall prosper in the

thing whereto I sent it. For it shall go out with joy and be led forth with peace.'

— Isaiah 55:10–12

The name of God is to be highly exulted, for God places great esteem on the words of His mouth above His name, and the son who was so close to His heart (King David) knew this. This is why the psalms sang praise to His Majesty – because He magnifies His word above His name **(Psalms 138:2)**.

Even Satan is scared of the truth; we know this is why his tricks are to confuse people and make them think the Bible is contradicting. In turn, most believers find it hard to read the Bible or to study or understand the scriptures; a dozen others who read the scriptures may not tread with care to study the words so that they know how to apply them. It is not enough to know the word of God. God is not interested in the words that we cram; rather, He is more interested in the words that will crown. We are crowned by the word once we become the word by the actions we take after hearing the word exactly **(James 1:22)**. Doing what the word says is how we can withstand Satan and tell him to get lost – 'I owe you not a thing.'

God wants us to use His word as our defence in every crossroads before jumping over the fence. Yeshua knew the right words to say to Satan when Satan went to tempt Him in the wilderness at the end of His forty days of prayer and fasting.

The tempter came to Him and said, 'If you are the Son of God, tell these stones to become bread.'

Then Yeshua answered, 'It is written: "Man shall not live by bread alone but on every word that comes from the mouth of God."'

Read **Matthew 4:1–11** and see how Yeshua commanded Satan with the word of God, which has already gone ahead of time for our use in times of need. Again, by the utterance of 'It is written', Yeshua used this as a point of reference to Satan each time He was tempted. After Satan saw that his time was up because the Messiah was functioning on the wisdom of the word, he backed off and left the begotten son of God alone on His mission to His ministry.

The word of God would always back itself up. This is the reason why we come across more than one verse in the Bible that would guide us into truth on a particular topic or subject that may be of concern to us or that we need reassurance on. Also, there are life testimonies of real biblical characters who have gone through what we may be experiencing. These testimonies are available for our referencing so that we may land on the assurance that the same God of yesterday is the same ancient God of forever and that His words never fades.

◯ **Praying in the Spirit** ◉

'Praying always with all prayer and supplication in the Spirit and watching thereunto with all perseverance and supplication of all the saints.'

— Ephesians 6:18

The word of God also teaches us through the help of the Holy Spirit and reminds us about what we've already heard from God: **'I will instruct thee and teach thee in the way thou shalt go. I will guide thee with mine eye' (Psalms 32:8)**. In this way, those who worship God should worship Him in spirit because He is the Spirit. All these guidelines are taken from the scriptures, so we are in line to receive results when we follow these guidelines. As such, we are also admonished to pray in the language of the Holy Ghost by speaking in tongues as the Holy Ghost is our intercessor.

Most of the time, there are a lot of things that go on in our life that pose as overly important. These things try to pull us from the presence of God, but even in such trials, this is when we should come into contact with God through praying in the Holy Ghost's language, especially when we don't fully understand the battles that we face or know where they are coming from. This is why the scripture says **(Romans 8:26)** that the Spirit helps our weakness and makes an intersection on our behalf when we don't know what to pray. Likewise, when we pray, we should listen to the guidance of the Holy Spirit so that we can do at ease the things that we have been created to do.

As the Spirit of God is the Holy Spirit that helps us to make intersections with God the Father, it cannot go wrong because it knows exactly what it wants us to pray on. It is also more beneficial for our spiritual and physical growth when we maintain this prayer method exercise. We are to pray to the Holy Spirit with faith in our minds even when we are in a fearful and toxic environment.

Mind Food: When fear seems to steal your voice and your sense of self in God, even if you cannot alter any word, keep still and try saying 'Holy Ghost' repeatedly in your mind to call on the presence of the Holy Ghost into your consciousness. Then look for a calmness within you and tap into the peaceful zone of the spirit where you can zoom in with the Holy Spirit. God has given us the Spirit of love, and love casts out all fears because that is the Spirit of God, and the Spirit of God is love.

- **2 Timothy 1:17 — 'God has not given us the spirit of fear.'**
- **1 John 4:18 — 'Perfect love drives out all fears.'**
- **Jude 1:20 — 'Pray to the Holy Ghost.'**
- **John 16:13 — 'The Spirit of truth would guide us into all truth.'**

◐ Obedience in Prayer ◉

It was through obedience that the servants were able to see water turn into wine (John 2:7–9). Had they stood and argued among themselves about what water had to do with wine, they would have missed out on being the first witnesses of the miracle performed by the Messiah. The almighty God has the capacity to deliver anyone whom He chooses to deliver. Therefore, when we have been led by the Holy Spirit to support others or comfort others, we should not worry about the provisions on the ground before stepping into obedience. My head is too small to comprehend how large God's capacity is, but I do not have too small a heart to contain His love and have the joy to serve Him.

I say to some people, *'When you have a message from God for the people of God, don't sit on it. Send it off at once because it will have an instant response, even if you cannot see an immediate response. In the Spirit, there would be a conviction that the angels of God have already put into action.'*

Merisha Meisha

However, while following instructions, we should learn to trust the Holy Spirit, for it is leading the way. Follow it thoroughly and remember – if in doubt, call on the Holy Ghost for a mysterious, supernatural intervention from heaven, for we must do the following:

> **'Trust in the Lord with all thine heart; and lean not unto thine own understanding. In all thy ways, acknowledge Him, and He shall direct thy paths.'**
>
> **— Proverbs 3:5–6**

It is in our obedience that we gain wisdom from God freely so that we can apply it easily to the issues of life, for what seems hard to others, we can obtain with ease as a result of our obedience at work, while disobedience puts a delay on our destiny. A quick response to the prompting of God almighty opens the closed doors that the enemy has shut against our lives to prevent the release of our open heavens, similar to when the master Yeshua told Simon to let down his net (Luke 5:4–5). With obedience, we work at a speed and come up with divine ideas that make people wonder where we get such ideas from because they themselves could not implement them, even with special aid.

Now when he had left speaking, he said unto Simon, 'Launch out into the deep and let down your nets for a draught.'

Simon, answering, said unto him, 'Master, we have toiled all the night and have taken nothing: nevertheless, at thy word, I will let down the net.'

Consequently, Simon's net was so heavy with the amount of fish caught that he could not pull the net up alone, which proves that obedience gives rest of mind and validates our relationship with the Commander.

Imagine two staff members employed by an employer. One staff member is always defiant, rejects works, and complains that extra working hours with the company do not reflect on their pay cheque. The other staff member accepts work tasks even if they are proven to be difficult and works outside the contracted working hours.

When an opportunity for a job promotion turns up for that company, my thoughts are in sync with yours. The staff member who complains will miss out on the opportunity to be promoted for the job and will possibly be fired and replaced, especially if they appear to be a liability to the company.

Mind Food: From time to time, check your obedience tick-off list if you want to keep moving forward in all areas of your life to prevent stagnation.

Imagine, as a child, if you had to ask your parents the 'why' questions, like a 2-year-old whenever they are instructed to do something. Now depending on how old you are and how close you want your relationship to be with your parents, if you ask 'Why?' all the time, you have to do as they advise all the time, and this behaviour continues into the adult stage. That relationship is not going to be a very intimate one. That parent–child relationship is going to be an adventurous one that will end up leaving the parent too exhausted to engage in the remaining things that should be enjoyed as a family because the time spent correcting the child has eaten away time for other creative family adventures.

God is quite austere in His ways, so let's not misunderstand this loving Father to love His children to death. To this degree, we must forego rebellious questions. As such, once we have heard the instructions right, we should avoid confusing our instant reactions with responding to prompt instructions so as not to slow down the hands of God, which operate on our behalf.

Check out the instructions and reactions of the people whom the Messiah healed during His ministry. He told them to go, that their faith had made them whole. Some, He told to pick up their beds and move, and others, He told to go and wash in a pool or so. Different people have different instructions because we come with different cases to present, so our sacrifice instructions are certain to be different.

'Whosoever has my commandment and keeps them is the one who loves me. The one who loves me will be loved by my father, and I too will love them and show myself to them.'

—John 14:21–23

Therefore, obedience is better than sacrifice (**1 Samuel 15:22**). The Master gave specific instructions to the blind beggar who was born blind. The instructions were for him to wash off the mud on his eyes in the pool of Siloam. The man was already healed, but his light was not turned on until he washed the mud off from his eyes in the water that he was told to take a rinse in (**John 9:6**).

When you delight yourself with God in obedience, you become His delightful son and daughter.

I am now learning to ask, 'What is it?' and wait for the Holy Ghost to lead me where to go next. However, if I have not heard clearly or understood the instructions properly rather than diving into the deep ends of the water, which would mean me leading myself and going by myself, I try to sit on my stool for a bit longer and wait for new inspiration from the Holy Spirit.

It is true that our obedience would be tested to see where our thoughts are focused on. Surely, the devil would come in through people to test us, and how often we worship God in our hearts would depend on how quick we are to follow His lead or fall off balance. The following quotes wherein God tests the minds and hearts of His people to see whether they adore Him are taken from the Bible. Rather than spend time murmuring in our minds, we can use the space in our hearts for meditation instead.

- **'Whatsoever things are of good report; if there be any virtue and if there be any praise, think on these things.' (Philippians 4:8)**
- **'Examine me, O LORD, and prove me; try my reins and my heart.' (Psalms 26:2)**
- **'The finning pot is for silver, and the furnace for gold: but the LORD trieth the hearts.' (Proverbs 17:3)**
- **'The LORD search the heart. I try the reins, even to give every man according to his ways and according to the fruit of his doings.' (Jeremiah 17:10)**
- **'Search me, O God, and know my heart: try me and know my thoughts.' (Psalms 139:23)**

God will recompense us in due time but not until after we have obeyed Him. However, delayed obedience is equal to disobedience.

◯ Command Prayer ◉

Yes, command that devil to get out of your case. Sometimes I just need to shut out the devil, as if I were deaf to him, especially when I find out the truth and discover that it is the devil that has been toying with me in the area I'm expecting a breakthrough in. It is not by our might or power but by the grace of God. As long as we understand our believer rights, we must take charge of full dominion over that situation and make the most of the power that God has given to us to cast out the demons. So we must use it in the right order as it is our right to do so.

Once upon a time, in 2017, I drank Coke in the daytime, but I noticed that through the night of that same day, I could not sleep. The following night, the same action was repeated. This time, however, I stood on my feet and shouted for the devil to flee, and he did. As I went back to bed, I slept for the number of hours I desired to rest for and was in good shape the following morning. I still drink Coke at least once a year if I want to but not more than twice a year, and I have not experienced such repeated performances as the one described above.

◯ Praying and Fasting ◉

'But we all, with open face beholding as in a glass the glory of the Lord, are changed into the same image from glory to glory.'

— 2 Corinthians 3:18

When the Holy Spirit of God begins to draw us nearer to God, it is because God wants to take us higher, but before He takes us higher, He will test us to see if we are ready for that position first before crowning us for the enthronement.

Prayer and fasting time is an intermediate time of waiting, just like Queen Esther knew the secret of waiting on God for an instruction. This is why she declared three days of fasting and praying for her and the Jews (her people) before going in front of the king to make a request. Even though this action cut her life short, the difference is that she first went before the King of Kings for direction before going in front of a mortal king to execute her plans that saw her opponent persecuted. **(The book of Esther is the seventeenth book of the Old Testament in the Holy Bible.)**

Prayer and fasting time is a time to be vigilant because this is a period when all manner of temptations come out from the woodworks. Some would try to push us over the edge or even paralyse our spirit, disabling our spiritual lives and rendering our spirits paralysed. This will cause prayer infirmity in the life of a believer so that they can give in to prayer and fasting. There is a crucial difference between when we are tempted by the Holy Spirit and when the devil tempts us. The Holy Spirit will tempt our faith in Him, while the devil will tempt our stand with God. One major difference that stands out is that when God tempts us, it leads us into wellness rather than into the well when Satan tempts us.

Imagine this scenario for a moment. Yahweh will give you instructions on when and where to pray; then He will leave it up to you to obey. Having heard this clearly, you will have to decide if you want to walk in full obedience or try to compromise the potency of the instruction. Now if you decide to use part of the prayer hour to go shopping as well as go to a totally different location from where you have been instructed to be at the time of prayer, you have not only led yourself away from God's guidance; you have also ignored all the gentle reminders of the Holy Ghost to put you back on track, along with leaving yourself naked for the tempter to gamble on your empty stomach.

As you move on with your day while minding your own business, a random person from the street bumps into you very abruptly and refuses to apologise, knowing fully well that they are at fault. Your natural response as a human being will be to lash back at that person, but you have your morals, which you are guided by. So you would normally approach this incident in an amicable way that will leave both parties not feeling dejected. However, suddenly, an anger you can barely grab and keep under control arises from inside of you, which now provokes you to decide to give this person what they bargained for just to prove that they must not mess with you. You backslide and end up insulting them, but just as you are about to leave their presence, you notice that your behaviour has made them feel pitiful and uneasy. Nevertheless, even if you notice the despair in their expression, you do not attempt to

25

show any form of remorse; rather, your blood boils over but this time with the feeling of guilt. You are not able to think through this until you get back home and in a calm environment, where you are able to reflect on your day.

While you're reflecting, a coin drops, and you are able to think through things properly. Can you now separate the test from the temptation?

Had your obedience been completed then, you would have been able to overcome or completely avoid the temptation of the devil in this period if it came in another form. If this had been a real scenario, God would have been testing the person's character to judge if they are willing to sacrifice their time for Him and obey what He had instructed them to do as a priority and within the time set. Meanwhile, the devil would have seen a gap in the window to tempt the character by pushing an innocent passer-by who is totally unaware that they have been used by the devil to cause the saint to sin and sink.

This is what happens when we leave ourselves naked – the devil slips in. We must try to remain in spirit when we are fasting especially and be fast to react yet slow to retaliate so that we don't fall into operating from the realm of the flesh, thereby dropping drastically from the supernatural to the natural just at the nick of time when we are about to receive a revelation from God.

In such a scenario, if played out in real life, the character of the believer who is supposed to be walking in obedience would demonstrate through their actions that they have lost some of their reasoning to judge whether the passer-by may have had a bad day or so, which warranted them to behave erratically. This is because they were taken over by the devil the minute they gave in to flesh. As a result, they fell to the sin of disobedience; hence, the spirit of God left them to fight for themselves because they chose to walk in disobedience and not divine guidance. Therefore, this character would have failed the test of obedience and fallen into the temptation of anger and un-forgiveness.

Another method that God uses to see where our hearts are is seeing if we would give Him all of our hearts while engaging in the fast. The Holy Spirit also expects us to share our food with others during this period. I have heard clearly from God a lot of times about giving, and I have gotten instant rewards, things I was not even expecting to receive, and some of the rewards are spiritual rewards and enlargement in that respect.

I know it's not so easy to give all the time because sometimes when I am starving for a particular meal and happily looking forward to indulging in that dish or snack, I hear God tell me to give Him that. By this, He means I should give my food to some other person who needs it more than I do and may not be in the position to afford a meal. You can imagine what my first reaction would be when I get such messages from heaven.

I try to plead with God to let me have my food this time around, but I don't get a 'Go on then. You can have it this time.' The response to my request is absolute silence until I obey, and even after obedience, I don't get an automatic response or a 'Well done, my child.' Still, I know that although my reward may not be always instant, there is a positive shift with my relationship with God just by obeying Him.

When we wait on God, the Holy Spirit takes our hands and guides us to the answer: 'I will instruct thee and teach thee in the way which thou go: I will guide thee with mine eye' **(Psalms 32:8)**. An example of how the supremacy of God searches all things and makes it possible for us to have things through the Holy Spirit, which moves around us, is a bit like the movie *Casper*. The major difference is that the Holy Ghost is real but unseen yet witnessed strongly within us.

In this way, Immanuel (one of the names of the Holy Ghost) knows where you go to most and what your interests are without requesting for your information to be stored on iCloud or on any technological devices to track you. Unlike these manmade methods, the Holy Ghost knows our thoughts, and when we choose to have a closer relationship with Him by involving Him more in our activities, the Holy Ghost will order our footsteps.

Waiting time can be an opportunity for our footsteps to be ordered by the Holy Ghost. In this manner, He ordains our day, and in so doing, He can arrange for someone to deliver items that would lead to our next breakthrough; such needs can be met in so many different ways and often offered to the person free of charge or sold at a giveaway price.

An example of this can be seen when you are fond of going to the library to use the space for your studies or research projects. Immanuel (the Holy Spirit) can orchestrate the librarian to walk past you with perfect timing with the book that you need. You don't even know it yet, but that is the book with the answers you need to solve the puzzles and resolve the issues that have been holding you backward.

In our waiting time, God gives us the answers to our problems at the nick of time when we rest on Him and do not allow the problems surrounding us to swallow us. Again, when we least expect it and at the nick of time, Immanuel sends our destiny helpers to cross paths with us and carry us to the next bus stop that leads to our final destination, or they can even take us straight to the point of dock.

So the Holy Ghost has no restrictions when it comes to reaching and locating whom He wants to save, but when we are saved, we are not just saved to be kept safe but also delivered from problems as lovers of God so that we can be problem solvers for other sufferers. God gives us the answers so that we can provide the answers for other people, along with bearing one another's burdens. In such a manner, He loads us with the goods so that we can offload the goods to others, making sure that we're the first to receive the treats and keeping us in the best position to absorb the benefits of having the aspirations of the Holy Ghost in our lives.

As we are first-time partakers of the answers to these issues, this puts us at an advantage of knowing the quality of what we carry. This encourages us to maintain attitudes as solution providers who mainly seek to find out how to resolve problems rather than constantly asking others for the answers. This is so that we can renew that grace as destiny helpers rather than use God for our personal gain and needs every single time without any reservations. The question to ask when we go to God in the instance of seeking divine guidance would be 'Show me, Holy Spirit – what is the way out? Now take me out. Take me out now.' If we get rescued all the time when we find ourselves in potholes without knowing how to get out, the day when we might get really stranded, it will be almost impossible for us to untangle ourselves from the potholes, which could be detrimental.

After we have overcome problems that we have already gotten answers for, even though we notice that the healing process has begun, there is still a period of waiting between the start of the miracle and when the miracle is completed. If we are consistently following the instructions given and we believe that we've been given the answers to the problems, when we see someone else who has the same issues and we are quick to help them out, God will miraculously hasten our healing or deliver us from those problems. At the same time, He delivers the person whom we have led to Him, shining the light of God upon them through the wisdom of God, given to us via the Holy Spirit. The Holy Spirit is constantly waiting for us to show up, so we have to learn to wait upon the feet of God for an answer.

> **'And therefore will the LORD wait that He may be gracious unto you, and therefore will He be exalted that He may have mercy upon you: for the Lord is a God of judgment: blessed are all that wait for Him.'**
>
> **— Isaiah 30:18**

There is a time for everything – a time to ask, a time to wait, and a time to receive. If we get everything we ask for in an instant, we will not learn anything from the experience of growing while we process where God is guiding us in the incubating stage. Waiting in the incubating stage is vital because if the process is hurried at all times, there would be zero growth. The goods will not be valued, and a product that we can hardly place a value on is as good as saying that the product cannot be vouched for.

God is deliberate with our growth, just like any natural parent would be deeply concerned if their 12-year-old is behaving with the mental capacity of a 6-year-old without any medical diagnosis as the reason for their malfunctioning. So our Father in heaven is also mindful and watchful over us in all areas of our growth, including our physical and mental growth.

The waiting period is also a testing period. The Bible mentions that our faith would be tried **(1 Peter 1:17)**. The Bible says that these trials will determine if our faith is genuine. It also suggests that it would be like fire passing through gold, so the outcome must be something worth much more than a million tonnes in gold as a soul is more meaningful and valuable to God than anything else that He has created in the world. So be mentally prepared for your flesh to be pruned and allow spiritual edification so that your journey with God will be elevated.

While waiting let's not forget to ask God to show us His ways so that we would follow Him, like when Moses asked to see more of Him in **Exodus 33:13: 'Now therefore, I pray, if found grace in your sight, show me Your way that I may know You and I may find grace in Your sight. And consider that this nation is Your people.'**

It is important that, while waiting, we believe that working in God's kingdom is a priority. There are so many people around us who are swimming through problems on a daily basis. These people are not strangers to us; they are people we live, work, and fellowship with and are a great opportunity to take advantage of this question in the completion of the task asked by the master Yeshua to Simon Peter, one of the disciples: 'If you love me, then put it to an effect by feeding my sheep' **(John 21:15–17; Matthew 6:16–18, 33).**

I have noticed that whenever I feel hungry when I am in the fasting and prayer season, it is because I am not engaging in prayers as much as I should. So when my prayer increases, my hunger diminishes because my spirit is being fed and satisfied with the presence of the Holy Spirit, and so it fuels my whole being to function without fainting.

The scripture below has really helped me a lot and has pushed me up the hill when I feel faint; I recite it, and it revives me to push on forward:

'But those that wait upon the LORD shall renew their strength. They shall mount up with wings like eagles. They will run and not get tired. They will walk and not become weary.'

— Isaiah 40:31

Prayer-Answering God

Are my prayers in the clouds and not reaching the heavens?

Has it not been written in Isaiah that God's spoken words would never go back to the heavens unfulfilled? So trust that when we pray, the most high, all-living God is committed to answering our prayers, but it is our faith that guarantees that our requests are met **(Isaiah 55:11)**.

I have observed some groups of persons waxing through multiple testimonies, while others are still holding onto prayer points for ages; likewise, there are some prayer points that I have held onto longer than anticipated, but God has granted me multiple instant miracles in between, holding onto these prayers being delivered to me. I may not always know why those other prayers are still pending. Even so, I get to witness God all over afresh each time I see the answers to my prayers because prayers answered announce the reality of God in my life, which reassures me that God remains a prayer-answering God who is too faithful to fail me.

Other times we may wonder if God is fair in His approach to responding to our prayers. This could be that when we are in desperate need for our prayers to be answered urgently, it skips our minds that God's timing is not ours. Apart from this, whenever we come closer to God, He never leaves us the same way as when we went to Him. Even if we may not notice the changes immediately, other people around us may notice these changes in our characters first and then mention it to us. This may surprise us initially because we are just becoming new versions of ourselves and have not fully become purified yet in areas where God is working on both our physical and other appearances. In all, the nearer we draw to God, the quicker He grabs the opportunity to cleanse us so that we are the edified versions of ourselves for the world to see, which we have been in His presence, therefore allowing all the glory to go back to Him as He takes us from glory to glory.

Our maker is more interested in seeing us purified and adequately capable of answering our questions and prayers. The question we should be asking when we go before God should not always be 'What can you do for me?' but should be 'What will you have me do next, o Lord?' Then we should wait for the instructions to follow. However, without purification, we would still be holding onto sin, which brings us down, thereby delaying the delivery of the answers to our prayers speedily. This does not mean that our prayers have not been answered; God is just waiting for us to do our bit before our requests can be portioned onto our plates.

At best, what really helps me not get frustrated after praying while waiting for answers is the attitude that I have adopted from Bishop David Oyedepo: whatever God has held back from me should be far away from me. What also helps me prevail after praying is that when I tap into the joy of the Lord, I imagine the raw hands of God delivering my prayers directly to me as I remember my previously answered prayers. Saying this does not mean the absence of tears when I pray.

See how Hannah prayed when she was expecting the fruit of the womb. Hannah did eat food and changed her containers after she prayed at Shiloh; therefore, change your containers after praying, especially if you are expecting the fruit of the womb like Hannah was, because the joy of the Lord is the confidence that we have to hold onto that God has given us victories even before we see the answers as He is certain to give us victory and complete our requests according to His will **(1 Samuel 2)**.

◯ Sharing Your Testimony ◉

Like the Samaritan woman at the well **(John 4:29)**, be quick to tell people to come and see what miracles the LORD has done for you once your prayers have been answered and your testimony delivered. A testimony shared is one multiplied, and the Bible says how else will they believe if they don't see the works of the Father in you, me, and our children for them to know that the LORD our God has given us to the world as signs and wonders? So let's not be tired of going out and reaching out to other people who are trusting God for a miracle, even if they have not yet yielded to the ways of the Lord, but through His wonderful works, this can draw them to repentance **(Isaiah 8:18)**.

Testimonies are prophetic; they speak of what we are waiting to see happen. They also increase our faith and keep our hope alive. After prayers, out come songs of assurance that our prayers have been heard. These signs keep us assured that our testimonies are sure because no one remains the same when they come before God. Even if we cannot see the full testimony yet, through the revelation of the word we have received from God, a transformation has already begun to take place in us, starting from our insides, thereby leaving our testimonies to be spoken boldly on the outside, just like in the case of Yeshua, the Messiah, as was recorded – **'He prayed the fashion of his countenance was altered, and his raiment was white and glistering' (Luke 9:29).**

With God, there are no coincidences but rather deliberations, with His delightful diligence granting us the desires of our hearts. This is one of the reasons why, when I hear the testimonies of others, I genuinely join them to celebrate as well as captivate the integrity of God's wonders at work in the lives of the persons.

As stated earlier, a testimony shared is one that is multiplied in the life of the teller and repeated in other areas of their

33

life as well as in the lives of those who hear and believe in it.
Sharing our testimonies is also a way of giving thanks to the almighty
Father but in the fashion of telling it to a multitude of people, saying,
'Once, I was blind. Now I can see.' Come and see for yourself, like a few
of the following testimonies.

In the book of Luke, as the master Yeshua was on His messianic duties in
Jerusalem, He healed ten lepers, but only one returned with a loud voice
to give thanks. He was made whole because of his attitude to gratitude,
while the remaining nine missed out on the perfection of the healing
because they did not return like that one leper. When you return with
your testimony, the Lord would put a seal on your testimony, and no
devil can steal it from you. The one who has seen your secret labouring
in prayer is the one who has chosen to reward you openly (**Luke 17**).

David, the son of Jesse and a lover of God, had his confidence boosted
when he remembered his testimonies of how God had helped him to
fight and defeat the lions when he was left alone with them in the forest.
This made him think of who can be against him and winning when God
is on his side. The young shepherd boy from Israel took up the challenge
to defeat Goliath, a giant war champion from Gath who was terrorising
King Saul and his people, knowing that no one would be able to win
against him in a battle. However, young David gained strength as he
remembered his testimonies, and God gave him the wisdom to kill a
huge figure with one stone from his catapult. After forty days of raving,
no one was brave enough to dare him in a fight (**1 Samuel 17**).

I have heard people spectating and debating on the testimonies of
others instead of respecting and appreciating what God has done in
the person's life and is about to do in their own lives if only they paid
rapt attention to the instructions and obedience for the testimony to be
manifested. Even the man who was born blind but was healed from his
blindness by the master Yeshua declared in front of the judges that once
he was blind, but now he could see, not caring if he would be persecuted
about declaring boldly that the master had performed a miracle on him
(**John 9**).

The nail on my left thumb has not grown all of my life as far back as I can remember. As a kid, I had never seen a full clear nail on this thumb right up to my growing-up years and beyond. As a kid, I never thought anything of it aside from telling a lie when asked what happened to my nail (it was jammed on the door by a careless adult).

Moving on, I became concerned as a teenager about my broken, never-growing, discoloured, smelly, dirty thumb. My phobia was more centred on the beauty perspective, so I hid my thumb whenever I was attracted to a boy, my opposite sex. This made me go to a medical consultant in England for a solution, notwithstanding that I had once gone through a surgical operation on the same thumb in Lagos State, Nigeria. Unfortunately, the dermatologist advised me that the whole vein of the nail was damaged, and the option I had was to amputate the thumb or live with it black and damp for the rest of my life. For me, this was not an option, but as there was nothing I could do about it, I was left feeling furious and terrified of the thought that on one hand, I would have to live with a routine thumb, and on the other hand, should the decay go further than my left thumb, there could be any kind of amputation in any part of my body.

Bear in mind that I had already had an operation on this same thumb, but I can only remember sitting awake in front of the surgeon who performed the surgery as I watched, numbed, on that faithful day. Still, I cannot fully remember the state of my thumb before this procedure. Nevertheless, it must have been in a terrible state which left it black, and although after the operation, the colour changed from black to brown, there was still a cut-off point of growth on this nail and a broken line that was visible. It had a way of preserving particles like a pit, and in turn, it smelled like a pit.

This disfigurement on my hand caused such a huge amount of embarrassment for me as I was growing up. I had passed the childhood stage of my life where I could tell a lie to save the day. However, over the years, I spent money affixing false plastic nails to cover up the damaged nail. Even though I was occasionally mocked in foreign languages by the nail technicians, I wore the shame of such mockery in disguise as if I had not been bothered by it. This persona was important for me to maintain to avoid being sensitive with people's comments because I knew I had to endure this for a short time so I could endure a better service on my next visit.

Trapped in a child's mind still, I never grew out of the lie that my finger had been trapped in the door by a clumsy adult. Apart from these nail technicians and people in my very close circles, no outsiders knew about the dead and smelly thumb that remained on my hand all of my life because I did a good job of hiding it – until the lockdown in 2020. God Himself stepped in on the nail and began supernatural work on it without me praying about it for a single day. The nail grew by itself without any cracks and completely dried up. As this miracle unfolded before my eyes, the Spirit of the Lord revealed to me that the pit that I had come out from was the pit I had dug myself.

Today God has rescued you from everything that is making you live a lie. Therefore, you are restored to live a prominent life away from the dark unto a place of light that God has prepared for you. Every pit that the enemy dug in any part of you, no matter how deep, has been discovered now, and you are recovered so as to fulfil the destined purpose that God created for you in the mighty name of Yeshua Hamashiach.

◯ **The Holy Spirit** ◉

We should allow ourselves to be guided by the Holy Spirit when we pray because it is constantly monitoring our thoughts with the consciousness of God in our hearts. For this reason, the Holy Spirit helps us to pray according to the will of God, for it knows our innermost thoughts and our outermost plans and motives. Therefore, we need the Holy Spirit to pour unto us the Spirit of God so that we can continue to pray according to the will of God, to avoid praying amiss, but the objective of our prayer point must be visualised in our minds.

'Praying always with all prayer and supplication in the Spirit and watching

**themselves thereunto with all perseverance
and supplication for all saints.'**

— Ephesians 6:18

It is in the interest and nature of the Holy Spirit to give us inspiration, but when we ask for its presence, it crowns us with an overflow of divine ideas and revelations of things yet to happen. In the same light, the Holy Spirit teaches us how to pray and acts as our middleman between us and the Father.

**'In the same way, the Spirit also helps our
weakness; for we do not know how to pray as
we should, but the Spirit Himself intercedes
for us with groanings too deep for words; and
He who searches the heart knows what the
mind of the Spirit is because He intercedes
for the saints according to the will of God.'**

— Romans 8:26-27

**'Because you are sons, God has sent forth
the Spirit of His Son into our hearts, crying,
"Abba! Father!"'**

— Galatians 4:6

◯ Dance Praise ◯

After we have prayed knowing that God has answered our prayers, we should offer the Lord a dance of praise to show the Sustainer that our faith and eyes are on Him alone. However, God Himself does not need to prove anything to us because He is too faithful to fail. Still, we need to prove to Him that we walk by faith and not by sight. This way, we are assured that the reality of our hope in God would soon be steering us, with our answers delivered, even as we praise and quicker than we anticipate.

I remember that sometimes, almost as soon as I begin to imagine something happening, the answer is already delivered to me just as I imagine it without me having to pray about it. I get it granted to me cheaply as a result of me having given praise to God. I think of all these miracles, and I begin to laugh at the so-called giants and all the gangs from hell that are trying to undo and steal my divine health and blessings to make the glory of God upon my life hidden. However, God, in His mercy, keeps showing up in my favour and lifts me up every time I get knocked down.

In a boxing ring, the winner could be the one who bleeds most and is wounded more, but remember this. When you get knocked down, it does not mean you're knocked out, so pick yourself up before the bell rings and try again, for there will always be God's hands to lift you up, even if you cannot see it. Just believe that you are lifted.

'Now faith is the substance of things hoped for, the evidence of things not seen.'

— Hebrews 11:1

'For we walk by faith, not by sight.'

— 2 Corinthians 5:7

Praise

In the world, they say, 'Fake it until you make it.' I say, '"Faith" it, and you will make it!'

I find myself laughing sometimes in the midst of conflict because certain mind tricks are clumsy, especially when the trickster leaves clues behind like mice droppings. Plus, just to confuse the enemy who's trying to be strong in my face, I laugh at the face of the enemy. Don't get me wrong here. I do cry from time to time, but it is rare for me to cry nowadays, which tells a different story about my days before now.

Once upon a time, I cried almost every day. In fact, some professionals kept the tissue box nearby, and some were quick to offer it to me as soon they saw the first tear drop because they knew I would soon be needing the mop bucket if care was not taken. I cried so often then because of not knowing the source of my pain because I was clueless as to the things of the Spirit. Nevertheless, I catch myself when I start crying, even when it hurts, taking my tears to God and dancing in front of the Most High, notwithstanding the tears rolling from my eyes down to my checks. Before I realise what's happening, I'm laughing hysterically, as if I'm being tickled by invisible hands, because I remember God's promises to me. Not one of the revelations I've received from God is said to give me a miserable end, not even upon my departure from the earth.

When we take the responsibility to praise God with every part of our being, we commit God's integrity to act instantly on our behalf. So make praise the smarter key to faster answers to your prayers. However, it is knowing how to praise God that will show us which key opens which door is determined for our breakthrough. Again, knowing how to praise God means our hearts are involved in praise and our minds are focused on God and God alone while we are praising Him so that we are not left stranded or frustrated in front of the door that is already unlocked but waiting for us to walk through.

If you have to push, push. Why stand in front of an open door when all you have to do is push? In the kingdom of God, nothing is done without a purpose. You are created for a purpose, so be encouraged and remain standing in faith. Hold on to what God has spoken to you about in secret because your open door is already unlocked if you believe it is. All you have to do is push slightly or even firmly, and God will make your entrance transparent.

Whenever I dance in praise in my room, I make sure the furniture is on the far end of the room so I don't have to care about anything else but myself and the Holy Spirit. This is different from when I dance in praise in public; I automatically keep my eyes closed so that people don't confuse my body movements and think as if I am entertaining them. Rather, I continue with my dance, and if they must gain my attention by the attraction of what I'm doing, even if it may seem odd to them or simply nice, I find a way to express the greatness and goodness of God in my life and also try to demonstrate that they too can tap into the joy of the Lord to improve their mental well-being and physical health.

In all, I pray in my heart that they see just a fraction of me and all of God around me and that by the exaggeration of my expression, I am too small to describe how big the wonders of God are yet how merciful and kind He has been to me. So if they can see this expression of my gratitude for who God is to me, how much more could He mean to them if they too can come a little bit closer to Him?

Celebrate God in praise to shame the enemy that is trying to see your downfall. There are several occasions when, almost immediately after I engage in a dance of praise, God grants me an instant miracle over something I have not even prayed for, and the Holy Spirit makes me know that that is the result of my praise; my miracle was delivered to me to shut the mouths of my enemies.

Mind Field

The power of engaging the mind in prayer is the most effective way of winning in prayer because the battles of life start from the mind of the person. It is what we entertain in our minds that we ascertain in any mountain or valley we approach. If you can win the battle in your mind, then you have won the fight before it becomes a war.

A biblical example to learn from when engaging the mind during prayer is seen in the woman with the issue of blood. She considered it in her thoughts: **'If I may but touch Him.'** After she touched the garment of Yeshua, other people heard how she had been instantly healed and then began to reach for the garment of the Master (**Matthew 9:20-22 and 14:36**).

'Casting down imaginations and every high thing that exalteth itself against the knowledge of God and bringing into captivity every thought to the obedience the Holy Spirit.'

— 2 Corinthians 10:5 (paraphrased)

'The bleeding woman' had this issue for twelve years, and even if she had spent all her money on physicians, she was not exempted from being stigmatised and stagnating in her community, but this embarrassment was brought down in an instant. She was attentive to the news that the Saviour was passing by and positioned her body to give herself both the mental awareness of how to reach for the garment of the Lord as well as the flexibility and balance that she needed to touch His garment in the midst of the crowd. Likewise, just by repositioning her mind and body for a touch, she received that power that the Master was carrying, which made the capacity that was operating on heaven's frequency flow into her blood stream and causing every disorderliness in her blood flow to cease at once.

'The light of the body is the eye: if therefore thine eye be single, thy whole body shall be full of light.'

— Matthew 6:22

It is up to you, how you want to have your expectations delivered to you, but I choose to say things the way I want to see them happen in my life. For example, I have identified that I have dyslexia, which makes my work not brought to my table at the time I would want it to be. However, I am not going to accept a joke that suggests I am stupid from any of my colleagues because in the midst of that task where I am organising my brain as to how to put things in order, I am already seeing my real identity unfold in my mind. I begin to see the Spirit of God merging as one with mine, for the Spirit He has given me does not make me timid but empowers me with the speed of the Holy Ghost and renews me with a sound mind daily, as cited in the Holy Book (**2 Timothy 1:7**).

I have a HTSBSH mentality: hear it, think it, see it, believe it, say it, and have it.

- ***Hear it (the word)***
- ***Think it (the word)***
- ***See it (the word)***
- ***Believe it (the word)***
- ***Say it (the word)***
- ***Have it (as the word says it)***

— **Merisha Meisha**

You first see what you want out of the word with your eyes before you see what you want in your hands. If it is a house, for example, you draw a picture of the building from your head. Then while you are praying, you begin to fill in the gaps in the picture with paintings from the word that you can cite. By the time you come into praise with this mind-set, you can already see the completed building in your mind, awaiting your arrival with the assurance that God will give you the bunch of keys to the house during that praise session. So you walk away knowing that the house is already yours and that it will be just a matter of time before you have it in the physical world.

Change the picture and take charge of your current situation. This house can be a missing body part or whatever else the challenge is. It is up to you to change the picture into the image you want to see in reality. This is my reality, and it always works, and even when it hasn't worked out my way, God never fails.

◯ Focused Prayer ◉

'Kill your distractions, or they will kill your time and delay your products from coming in the right season.'

— Merisha Meisha

The mind is the busiest compartment in the body yet the most solitary, filled with so many invited and uninvited guests; this makes it sound like a complicated place to be in if you can't see where you are going. For this reason, we are told to keep our eyes single so that our body can be full of light because the eyes of the body are found in the mind of man **(Matthew 6:22)**.

◯ Test Your Faith ◉

God will give us the test of sacrifice. This is not a bad thing because when God tests our faith, it is because He already has a better, brighter plan for us, so His tests are not to mislead us or make us afraid. God puts us through certain tests in life so that we can grow through giving up something that we really love because of the satisfaction it gives us. However, God will tell us to give it up for Him, especially if whatever we are clinging onto is detrimental to our spiritual life. The love that our heavenly Father has for us is unconditional; whenever evil is removed from us, He replaces it with an aspect of His nature and character.

God never tempts us with evil or with what He Himself has not given us the capacity to overcome. However, on dark days, our faith may be tempted by God to see if we would turn to Him for light in the areas where we encounter challenges. The test would be if we are looking to His word and promises as the only option for light because we should be looking unto Him alone as the author and finisher of our faith and as our only helping and hiding place, for at the entrance of His word, out comes light **(Hebrews 12:2; Psalms 121:2; John 1:5)**.

One of the fleshy pleasures that people enjoy but is a hindrance to the spiritual life of the children of God is masturbation. Yes! Masturbation. Masturbation is playing with oneself for sexual pleasure. The addiction to this act in one's life is one of the things that position an individual on the other side, far away from hearing the voice of God. Still, thousands of followers of God treat this deadly habit as if it is a casual matter or a fashion status because of the lack of understanding of this scriptural warning: 'What? Know ye not that your body is the temple of the Holy Ghost which is in you, which ye have of God, and ye are not your own?'

I am moved by the way the King James version of the Bible begins **1 Corinthians 6:19** with a question and closes it with another question. Consequently, I love the description in the Young's Literal Translation Bible version that refers to the body as the statuary of God, indicating that the body is a sacred zone, so we should neither tamper nor toy with it. Saying this, I am also aware that so many believers are likely suffering in silence while battling with this sin in secret. Some may say it is enjoyable and hurts no other person. There are numerous claims that masturbation is enjoyable, with supporting evidential statements from psychological experts that masturbation releases tension. However, the undermining and belittling feeling that arises from the body and mind is an after-effect of masturbation; it is shown by other forms of evidence that this leaves the person feeling lonely and depressed after masturbating.

Once the effects of masturbation are understood, the trauma that could later happen in our lives should the act lead to addiction and depression should encourage us to disengage ourselves from this pitiful activity. God, being so merciful, sends the Holy Spirit to be our comforter at all times, and as long as our hearts are still yearning to meet with the heart of God, God will want our spirits to merge with His. First, He purifies us so that we are one with Him so that when the Holy Spirit comes to visit us, He does not meet us at a time when we are toying with sexual immorality, either with ourselves or with a third party.

'Having therefore these promises, dearly beloved, let us cleanse ourselves from all

filthiness of the flesh and spirit, perfecting holiness in the fear of God. And let us work toward complete holiness because we fear God.'

— 2 Corinthians 7:1

'Choosing rather to suffer affliction with the people of God than to enjoy the pleasure of sin for a season.'

— Hebrews 11:25

A character in the Bible known as father Abraham had his faith for obedience when he was asked to sacrifice his son Isaac. Until God sent an angel to provide a lamb to rescue the boy, Abraham demonstrated total trust in God and was ready to take his son's life, having had a deep knowledge of God in that if He could have given him a son after waiting for this promise for years, the same God would provide an option that was better all round, both for him and the boy. In return, God blessed Abraham beyond his expectations and further than his eyes could see **(Genesis 22)**.

Patient while Praying

'Because thou hast kept the word of my patience, I also will keep thee from the hour of temptation, which shall come upon all the world; to try them that dwell upon the earth.'

— Revelation 3:10

'That ye be not slothful but followers of them who, through patience, inherit the promises.'

— Hebrews 6:12

Another area where we would be tried is in our patience. Patience is a very crucial part of waiting when we pray. While exercising patience in prayer, waiting is not the test. The test is our attitude towards waiting because the things we do while we wait, such as being joyful for others who triumph in the areas where we are waiting and trusting God for a turnaround/breakthrough, matter to God. On the other hand, God also weighs the contents of our hearts to determine if our words match our intentions; for example, are we congratulating people with our mouths but secretly, in our minds, are jealous of their success and testimonies?

Patience is also one of the characteristics of the Holy Spirit. So while our patience is being tested, it is also a lesson for us to adopt the habit of being patient with the people around us; hence, this is one of the qualities of God's character because He loves people. Equally, how much patience we render to others would determine how much love and understanding we have for others. Therefore, as God is the rewarder, He certainly rewards you when He sees you loving the things that He loves **(Galatians 5:22–23)**.

Abraham was again tested for his patience while waiting for baby Isaac to be born. The Bible records that Abraham was 75 years old when God told him that his wife, Sarah, would bear him a son who would come out of her own body. However, this promise was not fulfilled until twenty-five years later, when Abraham was 100 years old. While Abraham waited for this promise to be fulfilled, Sarah got impatient and led Abraham to enter her housemaid, Hagar, yet Abraham remained faithful, giving thanks and praise to God continually until he hosted the angels that triggered his blessings to be released.

Abraham remained faithful, praising God while he was waiting for the prophecy of his unborn son to come to pass. His attitude showed that he never took his eyes off God. However, when his wife brought on the suggestion for him to have a child with Hagar, it shows that he failed the test of waiting for God's way to be the only way for his promised child to come into his life because the prophecy mentioned that it would be his wife, Sarah, who would bear him a son and not his maid, Hagar. God is so merciful; we have seen this even in our own lives, in the ways that He gives us so many opportunities to retake certain tests in life, even if they come in different forms, because His ultimate goal for us is for us to excel in our pursuits on earth.

'Trials' is another term used instead of 'tests' in the Bible. They are also God's ways to measure if our faith would remain steady while we pass through life's trials, like He did for Abraham. Abraham passed the test of faith when he was asked to sacrifice his son, whom he waited for twenty-five years to be brought into the world through his wife, Sarah.

Abraham, having seen that God's word is more solid than a fauteuil for him to rest upon, tossed himself onto God's armrest, assured that he would be rescued by the Father should he hand his son back to the Father. Hence, through faith, Abraham reasoned with himself and concluded that even if he released Isaac to God, God would bring back Isaac from the dead for the full prophecy of God to be completed. Abraham was sure that God would raise Isaac back up because he remembered that God had promised him that it was through the son whom Sarah would bring into the world that a nation would be born.

Having judged God to be too faithful to fail, Abraham reasoned with himself; he then judged his own faith in God and trusted the process all throughout. Therefore, we are not only to allow ourselves to be tried by God; we are to also put ourselves through the test and judge God faithfully because He is too faithful to fail.

In the world, people are used to judging others but not examining themselves. This is why you hear a few people say, 'While you are pointing at someone else with one finger, there are four fingers pointing back at you, so check yourself.'

Accordingly, from the scriptures, we are given the tools for thought. In other words, Yeshua the Saviour mentioned how it is possible to pull out the speck from our brother's eye when we ourselves have failed to see the plank in our own eye. Why not remove the wool from one's eyes first? Then it would be easier to see clearly before reaching out to help pluck out the plank in the other person's eye.

Subsequently, know that all things work together for good for them who love God. When we are praying, it is more important that we maintain our faith in God by paying attention to our thoughts rather than allowing our thoughts to drift about the mountains that we've created in our minds, more so because our utterances are being measured by the substance of our hearts. The one who searches out all things (Holy Ghost) would be able to determine if we are praying and believing that God is a prayer-answering God who will deliver our answers to us in good time or if our thoughts are actually cancelling out our prayers with the doubts we have built up in our minds.

When I first started my journey of trusting myself in God's hands when I pray, I would listen to my heart, and if I heard any inner critics in contradiction to what I was praying, I would get scared and then stop praying. Then I discovered that I can pray against the doubts. I began to pray for God to heal my doubting mind. Today, when I pray and I pay attention to my thoughts, if any doubt pops up, I rebuke it instantly, and in so doing, I hear the contradicting thoughts go mute almost at once, thereby allowing me to continue with my prayers in peace **(2 Corinthians 13:5; (Matthew 7:3–5)**.

God's integrity is beyond my imagination. So for any test that God puts us through, He has given us the capacity to undergo it, but it is up to us if we want to pull through to the potential of believing God right through to the end.

The Word Test

'And take the helmet of salvation and the sword of the Spirit, which is the word of God.'

— Ephesians 6:17

'In the beginning was the Word, and the Word was with God, and the Word was God' **(1 John 1)**. This means that nothing can happen without the word of God because in the beginning was the word. God uses His word to rectify us, restore us, and redirect our footsteps if we are going down the wrong path in life because the word of God created us and therefore carries light.

'Thy word is a lamp unto my feet and a light unto my path.'

— Psalms 119:105

We should keep the word of God inside of us so that when the enemy, who is the devil, comes to test our faith to see if we are really the sons and daughters of the living God, we can let him know that the word of God is the sword that guarantees us our victory. Like the Master, let the devil know in the wilderness that it is written so he dare not tempt Him as He is the head of all principalities and powers.

'Study to show thyself approved unto God, a workman that needeth not to be ashamed, rightly dividing the word of truth.'

— 2 Timothy 2:15

'My people are destroyed for lack of knowledge: because thou hast rejected knowledge, I will also reject thee, that thou shalt be no priest to me: seeing thou hast forgotten the law of thy God, I will also forget thy children.'

— Hosea 2:6

'Therefore, my people are gone into captivity because they have not knowledge: and their honorable men are famished and their multitude dried up with thirst.'

— Isaiah 5:13

Having the word of God inside of us is key to building our faith, especially when we face spiritual warfare with the enemy to retain what is rightfully ours. For example, during prayers on behalf of our children whom the enemy wants to pull away from the ways of the Lord, we need to let the enemy know that our defence is the word of God, which has already been built inside of us through our engagement with the word, which is the Spirit of God itself. Then to silence him, we should vocalise that 'our children are the Lord's, and He only gives perfect gifts' **(Genesis 2, 12, 15–16; Galatians 3:5-7; Luke 1:26–36; Romans 4:11–12)**.

> **'But without faith, it is impossible to please him: for he that cometh to God must believe that he is and that he is a rewarder of them that diligently seek him.'**
>
> **— Hebrews 11:6**

What is on our minds is who we are constantly becoming, and whatever has our hearts is what we tend to worship instead of God. This is why God will want you to give up certain things that cost you a lot time yet are full of stress and empty promises, such as a dead-end relationship, exchanging such things for an hour of Bible studies with God. This can only bring more hope and assurance of a brighter future. An hour with God alone daily is not much if you consider what you will get in return when the revelations come pouring to you straight from heaven. In all, James puts it this way – consider it joyous when our faith is being tried, for we will surely receive our crown in the end as the Lord has promised it to those who have loved and kept his commandments **(James 1)**.

When you are word loaded, this means that you have downloaded the word in you, and when you have the word in you, it will easily jump out from your spirit when you are praying. To keep the fire burning, keep praying in the Spirit but capture the word in your mind and have the image of what you are praying about fixed onto your heart so that you can see it in your mind's eye.

◯ **Praying for One Another** ⦿

The word of God said the following in James 5:16 – **'Confess your faults one to another and pray for one another that ye may be healed. The effectual fervent prayer of a righteous man availeth much. And the expectation of the righteous shall not be cut off, and his desires shall be granted.'**

My prayer life was charged up when I heard Pastor Nicolas Udoh of Living Faith Deptford say in 2016 that it could be boring, praying for oneself all the time. Soon after I heard that, I began to pray for the people who were persecuting me in my vicinity, and before I knew it, God stepped in to restore peace in my surroundings.

We are admonished to pray for one another, but we should apply the same principles when we pray for ourselves and remember that when we pray, we are not only asking for provisions but also asking for solutions. Likewise, we are also thanking God in advance for meeting our requests even before they have been answered. Bearing this in mind, we should also remember that when we ask, we should expect a 'yes', 'no', or 'wait for it' response. If we are sensitive enough to pick up the instructions from the Holy Spirit while placing our requests, the frustration of waiting for instant results to our prayers would be lessened.

◯ **Let Us Pray Our Lord's Prayer** ⦿

◯ **Our Lord's Prayer** ⦿

Our Father who art in heaven, hallowed be thy name.

Thy kingdom come.

Thy will be done on earth as it is in heaven.

Give us this day our daily bread

And forgive us our debts as we forgive our debtors.

And lead us not into temptation

But deliver us from evil, for thine is the kingdom and the power and the glory for ever. Amen.

The Lord's Prayer is the prayer that Yeshua the Messiah taught us how to pray in **Matthew 6:9–13. Although this prayer has seven elements, it is divided into two sections only.**

Our Lord's Prayer, although prayed as a whole, is in two separate sections, with seven rules that govern our prayer life. Subsequently, the prayer is broken down into a sequence of two sections and categorised with seven prayer supplications in the order that we ought to pray in. The first part of the prayer is acknowledging God for who He is by exulting His name and also acknowledging that it is God whom we have come to, to pray to, in His holy name. This is so that we are praying to and with God in a communion that connects us via our prayers, which means that when we pray to God, by the confessions of our spoken or meditated words in our hearts, we also have to wait to hear from God by listening for His directions, lead, and/or instructions. The second part admonishes us to lay down our supplications in the order that is presented to us, to intercede for one another while specifying our requests for one another. In other words, the first part is from us to the Father, for the Father. Then the second part is, again, to the Father from us but for us.

There are seven rules/petitions that we bring to the Lord when we pray the Lord's Prayer. These seven components remind me of God's creation of the world and that He is a God of order. Remember when He founded the world. First, He discovered the world; then He created the world to become what it is now because before the creation, the world was full of great emptiness, and from nothing, He turned it into something spectacular **(Genesis 1:2)**. Everything the Lord created, He saw that it was good:

'And the earth was without form and void; and darkness was upon the face of the deep. And the spirit of God moved upon the face of the waters. And God said, "Let there be light": and there was light.'

He said 'Let there be light' so that He could see the process of His creativity, which brought about the formation of the earth that was without form. God called forth light before other things that He created, which were spoken into existence, so that He could see and admire His creation. In other words, the word of God is in the order that it was spoken, starting with 'light', which gave birth to the formation of the earth, which was empty.

God created the world for six days, and on the seventh day, He rested. The seventh day is inclusive in the sequence of days included in the creation process of the universe. The significance of the seven elements of the Lord's Prayer is linked with the seventh day of God's creation of the earth, and His resting is reflected upon, with God being a God of order. The number seven, however, has significance for appearing in the Lord's Prayer, having being mentioned in Genesis for the first time. As well, the world runs on a seven-days-a-week basis for our consideration that there can be at least a prayer line for each day of the week.

The Lord's Prayer is already defined so that when we are praying, we are praying in a way that is accepted by God and understood by us as our prayers are our direct communication to God almighty. This means that the order that we ought to pray in is important so that our prayers can manifest into results with testimonies that will advance both our spiritual lives and our physical lives. Still, the whole essence of the Lord's Prayer is to encourage us to replicate what the Messiah did during His walk on earth so that we too can make good disciples within our communities.

'Verily, verily, I say unto you, He that believeth on me, the works that I do shall he

do also; and greater works than those shall he do because I go unto my father.'

—John 14:12

'If ye love me, keep my commandments.'

—John 14:15

Our Father Who Art in Heaven, Hallowed Be Thy Name

The almighty 'I AM that I AM', the all-holy God, is first our God; then He becomes our father when we have accepted and remained in His ways. When we call God our Father, we connect with Him as our Father through His Spirit, which makes our words to Him relatable and not just empty words. Our heavenly Father knows our needs, but just like our earthly fathers, our Father who art in heaven wants us to come closer to Him by remaining with Him through our prayers as this is our communication link with him. So when we say **'Our Father'**, we personalise this to affirm our stand with God; then God draws us even nearer and hears us. He hears our cries, feels our pain. When we are hurt, He is hurt too, and it pains Him when our enemies come to harm us. He defends us and curses things that curse us; just as any natural father would nurture his children, God does so for us, His children, too.

We, His children, are all united to God through our spirit to His Spirit, so when we pray, we pray to God the Father, God the Son, and God the Holy Spirit. We submit to our heavenly Father when we call on His Trinity and Supremacy. As well, we praise and worship His name just like the Lord God almighty Himself has told us to do repeatedly throughout the scriptures. He gave many examples of how most biblical characters like David, **Isaiah**, and even Yeshua the Messiah Himself showed us how we should give reverence to God in our praise.

'For it is written, "'As I live,' saith the Lord, 'every knee shall bow to me, and every tongue shall confess to God.'"'

— Romans 14:11

'Lord, you are my God; I will exalt you and praise your name, for in perfect faithfulness, you have done wonderful things, things planned long ago.'

— Isaiah 25:1

We say 'who art in heaven' because we are acknowledging that God is a resident in heaven, although His presence is with us on earth. He abides with each and every one of us because of His sovereignty. Again, 'heaven' is announced to reinforce our hope of knowing that as the children of God, we are called into heaven to be with Him eventually at the end of time as it is our final destination. This is why we should walk in love with one another so that our destinies leading to the place of holiness with God will not be cut off.

We start the Lord's Prayer by acknowledging the Father, who is God almighty, by consciously calling him 'our Father'. We call Him into our presence, and then we add 'hallowed be thy name' to salute the holiness in His name. God the Father is a Father to all of us, and we should all be praying in this manner and remain connected to Him not only during prayer time but always. He is our Father who hears our cries and feels our pain; when we are hurt, He is hurt, and when our enemy comes to harm us, He comes to our defence and curses those that curse us because of the love that He has for us. He feels our emotions; just like our natural fathers feel emotional towards our well-being, our supernatural Father feels the same emotions that we feel but releases our angels in human form to come to our aid. We, God's children, are all united with God through the Spirit of God, and we pray to God the Father, God the Son, and God the Holy Spirit, so when we call on our Father, we are calling on God's Trinity and Supremacy.

God is a God of order, and we link this with His creation of the world and the Lord's Prayer. The seven elements of the Lord's Prayer have significance in relation to the seven days of God's creation of the earth and resting. On this note, notice that the order in which God created the world unfolds with the events of His different creations from day to day. Likewise, this orderly way of presentation is seen in the way the Lord's Prayer is presented to the disciples in **Matthew 6:9–13**.

Thus, in the Lord's Prayer, we say the following:

- **Our Father** — We are united with our heavenly Father via the Spirit, which He put inside us during the creation, but this Spirit is only activated when we acknowledge it; it then goes into work for us with its supernatural ability but by our superintendence.
- **Heaven** — Our place to be eventually is heaven; otherwise, our walk with God here on earth would be pointless. However, to experience His glory even while on earth is by living a lifestyle of total wholeness in our bodies with peace in our minds. It is in the way of living up to heavenly beauty on earth because that tranquillity from heaven is transferred to us here on earth.
- **His Name** — We have to first recognise that God is holy and that His holiness is capable of cleansing our iniquity. This means that God does not need anything or any person in the whole universe to make Him holy, but we need God to make ourselves holy as He is and has called us to be. Therefore, we should salute the Holy name of the almighty as we concede that He is the only true almighty God for the reasons we have come to seek His presence.

Thy Kingdom Come

'Thy kingdom come' has been demonstrated by our Lord and Saviour Yeshua, who expanded His ministry by going from one community to another, spreading the good news of the kingdom of the Father that is yet to come. In doing this, Yeshua went about from town to town, teaching people how they should be living with one another in preparation to come into God's kingdom. In addition to this, some biblical characters have left us with many testimonies, and their own experiences of the reality of the Messiah on earth is proof which should propel us for the second coming of the Messiah.

⊙ Thy Will Be Done on Earth as It Is in Heaven ⊛

We ask for God's will to be done in the way that it is in heaven, but what is the will of God for us on earth? The following scripture paints a picture in my mind: **'Beloved, I wish above all things that thou mayest prosper and be in health, even as thy soul prospereth' (3 John 1:2)**. This portion of the prayer alone covers both my physical health and my mental health, which gives me the reassurance that my health is secured in God's hands; we ought to pray for one another with this scripture reference, especially as this is the way the Messiah taught us to pray, and God always honours what He ordains.

God's will is for the world to be healed with His word so that our wellness is established on earth for those of us who would believe. This is why He gave us His only begotten son **(John 3:16)**. If you have ever wondered why the world is in such destruction if God loves the world, the answer is in the fact that men have abandoned God's ways and gone on their own ways, away from God's leading. God wants us to pray for one another so that we can grow together in faith and bond closer as a people to overcome the trials that lie ahead of time.

We should also pray for one another so that we can be equally prosperous, but to be this way, we have to become as selfless as Emmanuel was and still is. Saying this, I am aware that most people, even believers (sons and daughters of God), most times misunderstand the meaning of prosperity, hence concluding that for one to be prosperous is not a good thing. They omit that one can be prosperous in health as well as wealth and family growth but especially with an individual's well-being.

This ignorance and lack of understanding of the core essence of wealth and the reasons why God makes a man rich keep some believers as beggars or impoverished for a lifetime when they could have gained wealth and advanced the kingdom of God with the knowledge that a man is enriched for the welfare of his nation; this is the reason why God puts financial blessings upon a man.

As a matter of fact, I first need to be prosperous in my health before I can be prosperous in my wealth; **3 John 1:2** is a good reference to touch and hold onto when it comes to reminding God in our prayers about one of His promises to us on our health and wholeness benefits for being in the same body with the Holy Ghost. My soul sits in my heart, which is the centre of my mind, which is the source of my mental health. So if I don't prosper in this area of my life, I am unable to achieve my goals in life or accomplish my God-given assignments and projects in the mental health sector.

As believers, we do not acquire wealth for the self but because of other indigents around us, which means that when God blesses us, He uses us as an avenue to be a source of blessing to others in our community, but blessings are not limited to financial uplifting only. We can be blessed with so many different gifts and talents that can be used to bless others around us. For example, praying for your family members and going to the hospital and praying for the sick to be healed is as good as blessing others, most especially when they walk into wholeness as a result of your prayers.

◯ Give Us This Day Our Daily Bread ◉

God wants us to ask Him and remind Him of the things that He has promised to us. Hence, we come asking for God to give to us what He has promised us because He already said that He has given us our daily benefits, *but what are these benefits and things that we are asking from God for ourselves and other people?*

God's provision is sufficient enough to sustain us right from the day we are born. Some may think this statement is impossible, but think of the natural resources in the many counties across the nations of the earth that are being mismanaged by greedy government systems which have kept millions of people impoverished in the world. Here, it is easier to blame God for some, while others keep the faith.

The story of Elijah reveals how God provided for Elijah supernaturally with a flock of ravens and spoke out boastingly about taking care of us; this is because He can do and has done so. After all, was He not the same God who fed our fathers in the wilderness with manna from heaven, and is He not the one who is still sending us rain from heaven to this day **(Matthew 7:7–8; Isaiah 43:26; 1 Kings 17:6; John 6:49; Leviticus 26:4)**?

The understanding of asking when we pray is in knowing that God's provisions for us are sufficient, but we must ask to be given that which is extraordinary, outside of what grace gives us daily, from the supernatural realm to our natural form. Notice the word 'ask'. God wants us to ask, not to worry but to ask; worrying triggers anxiety, which is not in the nature of God. On this note, we are to make our requests known to God, and the Holy Spirit would assign our angels to be put into work on our behalf.

Do not worry about your daily bread and needs; God fed the ravens in **Luke 12:24 and in Matthew 7:9–11**. In verses 7 and 11, see the metaphoric description illustrated to understand that God wants us to come to Him and ask of Him what we need:

> **'Or what man is there of you, whom if his son ask for bread, will he give him stone? If ye then, being evil, know how to give good gifts to your children, how much more shall your Father which is in heaven give good things to them that ask him?'**

Forgive Us Our Debts as We Forgive Our Debtors

'Forgive us our debts.' This supplication requires that we forgive others who have offended us first before we can ask God to forgive us our sins. This way, we are not hypocrites with our relationships to man and God, so we should be mindful that when we are asking for God to show His mercy upon us, we must be willing to forgive others and demonstrate this forgiveness to them with both our actions and our words.

In Isaiah 1:18, the Lord said, 'Come, let us reason together: though your sins be as scarlet, they shall be as white as snow' (paraphrased). The lack of forgiveness would hinder our prayer life, which would adequately affect our relationship with our creator because when we pray, we are communicating with God, and a good relationship needs transparency, not pretentiousness. As such, God sees the heart, so it is to our advantage that we practice forgiving ourselves first so that we can forgive others who offend easily even before the offence arises.

When you show others that you are capable of forgiving them no matter the offence, you are giving them a gift that would heal their soul. At the same time, you're healing your soul too as well as opening up a window that enables those whom you have forgiven to practice forgiving others and themselves. By practicing forgiveness, you also give Jehovah the room to defend you when others offend you and for Him to expose and dispose your enemies so you don't need to fight anyone in retaliation to the offence they might have caused.

> **'Did He not say: "Be still and know that I am God"?'**
>
> **— Psalms 46:10**

◯ Lead Us Not into Temptation ◯

> **'And He said, "That which cometh out of the man, that defileth the man. For from within, out of the heart of men, proceed evil thoughts, adulteries, fornications, murders, thefts, covetousness, wickedness, deceit, lasciviousness, an evil eye, blasphemy, pride, foolishness. All these evil things come from within and defile a man."'**
>
> **— Mark 7:20–23**

'Lead us not into temptation.' Temptation is what pushes us into sin and to covet what does not belong to us, but we are tempted through the thoughts that are injected into our minds first before the outcome of the temptation is manifested in our actions. This is why it is encouraging for us to pray for the spirit of discernment so that we can judge the things, people, and places that we should stay away from and also what not to say to whom and when to say what. Hence, when we fall into temptation and offend our fellow human being or sin directly against God, we should always be watchful as well as prayerful. In **Luke 22:31**, Peter was told by Yeshua that the devil was looking for which one of the disciples he could destroy with his vicious temptations. Again, in **1 Peter 5:8**, a reminder to be aware of the devil is highlighted because as this scripture warns, be on guard as the devil is **to and fro** like a lion looking for who to tear down with his afflictions.

Yeshua tells Peter in the above verse that He has prayed for him so that his faith does not grow faint. Following this, the scripture is painting a picture of how important it is that we pray for one another. Apart from praying for one another so that we don't fall into temptation, we are to take conscious and deliberate actions in training our hearts to be able to sieve the ants away from the sugar because not everything that seems good on the outside is good for our insides.

'Keep thy hearts with all diligence, for out of it are the issues of life.'

— Proverbs 27:19

The prayer of 'lead us not into temptation' is similar to the prayer of 'forgive us our sins' because they are both prayers of mercy. In this prayer, as sons and daughters of the Most High, we are asking our Father to grant us mercy and not allow us to fall into any holes dug up by our enemies. This way, we are depths away from falling into temptation and are delivered from the hands of the wicked ones in our midst. Still, even if it takes the mercy and favour of God to redirect our steps, we have to submit ourselves to Him through prayers and to bind us in His grace.

Some may ask, 'If His grace is sufficient enough for us, why do we need to ask this in prayer so that we are led away from temptation?'

When we ask God to show us those things about us and around us that are bringing us into a sinful nature, it is so that we can avoid them by His grace. We need to ask in advance because temptations come in different forms all around us. They also come with different traps that the enemy has set for us to trip over, even those in our minds, which is where the worst offence is committed and crimes are premeditated. So the prayer of walking away from temptation should not be underestimated; likewise, the offences that are the results of these temptations should not be underestimated either.

For example, someone can be tempted into making a hateful comment to somebody else, but the sin starts with them being jealous of the person before the hate speech is spoken to offend the other person. The whole event begins from the heart and, depending on the maltreatment, may end up making someone else feel depressed if they are already struggling with low self-esteem.

Interestingly, jealousy is a trait of the devil because he envied and still does envy everything that God created. However, because we are children of God, we lean towards our creator to cast out our secret sins from our minds so that we can overcome these temptations rather than fall more into temptation. Therefore, the scripture says, **'Submit yourselves to God. Resist the devil, and he will flee from you' (James 4:7)**.

◐ Deliver Us from Evil, for Thine Is the Kingdom and Power and Glory ◑

'Deliver us from evil.' We ask God to deliver us from the hands of Satan and those evil principalities that afflict us and cause us to sometimes fall out of faith and doubt if God's promises are real. These doubts are easier to filter into our minds when we are in pain caused by these afflictions. So for us not to give up hope and to keep on believing what the word of God says, we should pray endlessly that God deliver us from the hands of these evil principalities that are constantly in a spiritual battle against us to cease destiny or cause untimely deaths and stop us from fulfilling God's purpose in life, for the issues we face in life are not the seen battle.

'We wrestle not against flesh and blood but against principalities, against powers, against the rulers of the darkness to the world, against spiritual wickedness in high places.'

— Ephesians 6:12

When we ask God to protect us, we should also wait to receive His protection. Some of the things that God will give us are some of the things that He has already prepared for us in advance. However, in prayer, there is a waiting period to hear what God is directing us to do or how to be for that prayer to be fully answered – testimonies delivered in our hands. Some of the examples of praying for God's protection are noted and have already been seen in the lives of some biblical characters, such as in the life of David. This is a fine example to mirror when it comes to praying for mercy and protection **(Psalms 23)**.

The most powerful prayers are the ones taken out from the word of God and given back to God: 'Father, you said it here, and this is what you will do if I do this.' Another powerful way to get our prayers answered is by going back to God and reminding Him of what He did for someone else in the same area we are entrusting Him with for a breakthrough.

By praying for others, we are also praying for ourselves, so by praying for others with understanding, you are investing in your own life also, and this is another powerful way to get God to answer our prayers with speed. In all, the most effective way to get God committed in our prayers with speedy answers to them is when we depart from a sinful nature by being authentic with our repentance from sins.

The last one is for us to meditate daily on the word of God until we see ourselves becoming what the word of God says. This way, when we need to pray, we will not be searching for words to communicate to God with; rather, we will use the word that we know already, which God has already spoken to us in advance in the scripture, reminding us of revelations. This is why it is important to know God's written words – because it is the word that we know that God will speak back to us, and this is what will build up our faith to receive more revelations and instructions from our Lord, the King of Kings, our God almighty and heavenly Father.

'When your words came, I ate them; they were my joy and my heart's delight, for I bear your name, LORD God Almighty.'

—Jeremiah 15:16

When you build your faith up, you can face the battle and defeat Satan with the word, knowing that God is the one fighting for you, but you have to open your mouth and say the word because that's what punches the devil down: **'So then faith cometh by hearing and by hearing the word of God' (Romans 10:17)**. Therefore, the word of God is what you hear and understand. The word is what you can use to cast out the devil when he comes with his accusations anytime in the day or night so that again, the battle is won, and all the glory goes back to God, for if it was not for His sent word, that battle would have swallowed us up, as the enemy intended.

'Study to shew thyself approved unto God, a workman that needeth not to be ashamed, rightly dividing the word of truth.'

— 2 Timothy 2:15

Chapter II

THE TEN COMMANDMENTS OF GOD TO MOSES

Ten Commandments

**'Now therefore, if ye will obey my voice
indeed and keep my covenant, then ye shall
be a peculiar treasure unto me above all
people: for the earth is mine. And ye shall
be unto me a kingdom of priests and an holy
nation. These are words which thou shalt
speak unto the children of Israel.'**

— Exodus 19:5–6

The **Ten Commandments** have the key that can change the world
to become the way God desired it to be at its creation so that we would
live without struggle but in peace with one another. However, human
nature, since we are formed out of the seed of Adam and Eve, is sinful

because of disobedience to God's guidance. Hence, God sends prophets out to the world to deliver the message of repentance, which should be to reconcile men back to Him; as well, He raises teachers to teach the word of faith, which is the life of God.

Moses was the prophet whom God used to deliver the Ten Commandments to the people in **Exodus 22:2**. Here, Moses met with God (I AM) in the burning bush, where God appeared to him and unfolded His ministry to him. God then gave a set of instructions to Moses called the Ten Commandments, which are the covenant that He drew between Him and His people of Israel – *but who are 'His people'?*

> *'God declared that the Israelites were His own people, and so . . . they must listen [to] and obey God's laws. These laws were the Ten Commandments, which were given to **Moses** on two stone tablets, and they set out the basic principles that would govern the Israelites' lives.'*

> — **BBC** (www.bbc.co.uk>history>moses_1),
> **6 July 2009**

It will be interesting to carry out a brief search on the 'original Israelites' whom God is talking to and about to this day so that God's instructions will not be misconstrued, especially by the people whom they are meant for. With this in mind, other people who return to God through salvation are also taken in as the children of God, but God is more upset when those He classifies as His children disobey Him, as He was when the Israelites had done so.

'The earth is the Lord's and the fullness of it thereof: the world and they that dwell therein.' This scripture, among many others, is one of the ways God is sending an invitation to anyone who wants to accept His ways to come into His kingdom and abound therein after he or she has accepted salvation. In the book of Galatians, Paul says, **'So in [the] Messiah, you are all children of God through faith; all of you who were baptised believing in the son of God**

have clothed yourself with Yeshua. Therefore, there is neither [Jew] nor Greek, there is neither [bound] nor free, there is neither male nor female: for ye are all one in God through Yeshua' (paraphrased) **(Psalms 22:1–10; Galatians 3:38).**

Once you've found out that you are whom God is talking to, pay attention to what God is saying and be mindful to do as He has spoken for you to do so that the destruction that comes on those who disobey does not come upon you at the end of time and so that your salvation can be preserved. Obedience to God's instruction will not only secure your destiny but also secure that of generations to come, like that seen in the experience of Noah, when he listened not to men and built the Lord an ark, even when almost the whole of his city laughed at him. He focused on the task and was merited on its completion, and in so doing, the lives of his family were not truncated by the floodwaters.

The first commandment God gave to Moses out of the ten is that we should not have any other god apart from Him. The 'I AM' already knows that there are other gods that were created by the hands of men for themselves to worship instead of worshiping Him, but they are not our God as there is no other God but the almighty creator of the universe. This is why they are called gods and are created by the hands of men. **Isaiah 2:8–9 reads, 'Their land is also full of idols; they worship the work of their own hands, that which their own fingers have made. And the mean man boweth down, and the great man humbleth himself: therefore, forgive them not.'**

Unfortunately, the children of God want the blessings of Abraham to be 'mine' and for the double riches added to Job to be the same portions given to them, but how many of us are really willing to obey like father Abraham did and judge God as faithful like Job did because the scripture records that Abraham retained the promise of God through faith? This is referenced in **Romans 4:20: 'He did not waver at the promise of God through unbelief but was strengthened in faith, giving glory to God and being fully convinced that He that had promised He was also able to perform.'**

In the case of Job, God restored him and doubled everything he had lost because even in his affliction, he focused on God and prayed for his friends. Job looked unto God for help, and even when his friends accused him of having done wrong or sinned against God as a result of his affliction, Job forgave and prayed for them. Also, when his wife told him to curse God and die so he could be free from his hellish life at the time of his suffering, Job continued to look unto God until his help came from heaven. We can read about Job's defence of God's faithfulness in **Job 2**.

> ### 'My help cometh from the LORD, which made heaven and earth.'
>
> ### — Psalms 121:2

Like the Lord's Prayer, the Ten Commandments are divided into two sections. The first four commandments are concentrated on our love for God, while the last six commandments are concentrated on our love for our fellow human being, making love the greatest aspect that governs the Ten Commandments of God. The Bible said, **'The children of God are manifest, and the children of the devil: whosoever doeth no righteousness is not of God, neither he that loveth not his brother.'** In this respect, the love of God is of love, for God is love. This forms the first commandment, the greatest commandment. Yeshua said, **'Thou shalt love the Lord thy God with all thy heart and with all thy soul and with all thy mind.' The second part is 'Thou shalt love thy neighbour as thyself'** (Matthew 22:37, 39).

Throughout the Bible, we read different scriptures talking about love and how it conquers all challenges. I have written about how you can tap into the power of love to overcome obstacles in my book *Every Mind Matters to Messiah*.

(I)

◯ I Am the Lord Thy God; You Shall Not Have Any Other Gods before Me ◉

Creating a hierarchy of other things over God's instructions is prioritising these other things as important over God's things. Instead of obeying the Ten Commandments by doing as the commandments tell us to do, this rule is abandoned, and rather, the culture of idolising people and pastors is adopted in our behaviour as normal. What the section of this commandment is telling us is that we should serve God with all of our time, avoiding everything that demands the use of our time solely on it and has the potential of removing us permanently from the presence of the LORD. We should create time to have a fulfilled life all round, at the same time making sure that we have made time for the things that matter to us most, especially our spiritual life, which is designed for our edification.

> *'Putting God first may sound ridiculous, but it is the only way I am sure not to be ridiculed by the outcome of my growth.'*

> **— Merisha Meisha**

(II)

◯ Thou Shalt Not Make unto Thee Any Graven Image or Bow to Them ◉

Again, creating a hierarchy of other things over God's instructions is prioritising these other things as important over God's things. This practice is compared to putting graven images before the things of God. Instead of obeying the Ten Commandments by doing as the commandments tell us to do, this rule is abandoned, and rather, the culture of idolising people, pastors, and/or the self is adopted in our behaviour as a normal way of living.

Who is your God? My God is the 'I AM'. We should pay careful attention to this bit of the commandment as it requires our commitment. Although it's a reminder of the first commandment, the difference is that this commandment totally forbids us from worshiping any other image in any shape or form:

> **'Thou shall not make unto thee any graven image or any likeness of anything that is in heaven above or that is in the earth beneath or that is in the water under the earth.' (Exodus 20:4)**

Imagine God the omnipotent in a box. This would be limiting God's ability in one's mind because one's attention is given to the image that is carved with the hands of man. Then worshiping this image instead of devoting the time to serve the creator of men is like worshiping one's self, so there is no wisdom in this act.

Worshiping other images instead of God also displeases God because God created us in His image. We are to honour this as believers so that we can avoid recreating God according to our own perceptions of what God is rather than who God is, which will adequately reduce the comprehension of God's sovereignty in the mind of the idol worshipper. See what the LORD is saying in **Isaiah 29:13:**

> **'Wherefore the Lord said, "Forasmuch as this people draw near me with their mouth and with their lips do honor me but have removed their heart far from me, and their fear toward me is taught by the precept of men."'**

This indicates that we must search for God with our whole hearts from the words that He has spoken and were written by His prophets, like Isaiah, which were encoded in the Bible for our reference to study the mind of God. We can learn to worship Him with our bodies, mouths, and hearts for the fulfilment of the scripture and our enthronement.

We begin to hear what is being said to us clearly as soon as we discover who we really are in Christ our Saviour, and if we are attentive, we will perceive God saying to His people, 'Look up to me alone as your ultimate source for everything, not unto pastors, prophets, bishops, or pop stars because in the days of calamity is the "I AM" you will ever need to get you through and out of it.' Having said that, the reality is that people are lost before they are found through salvation, but faith in God does not come by salvation alone; it comes with believing as a believer, just like Job did believe to trigger the raw hands of God that multiplied his blessings.

(III)

◯ Thou Shall Not Take the Name of the Lord Thy God in Vain 🌐

Do not take the name of thy LORD in vain. Do not say the name of the Lord in a common manner. Do not swear before or after the name of the Lord. **Does this make you think?**

The name of the Lord is to be feared in love and adored in praise as it is our strong tower. Imagine if your surname was mentioned after every joke or was repeated as an exclamation anytime you made a vocal expression. If this becomes the case, I'm certain one will take deliberate action to forbid others from using their name in such a useless manner. This is an illustration of how the name of the Lord God almighty can be used in vain when we make remarks such as 'Oh my GOD!' during conversations where the subject does not warrant God's name being involved in it and is not related to godly matters.

Besides the above, as children of God, it is important for us to be mindful of how we present ourselves to the world as others are watching us. Because we are the light, we are to show good examples for them to follow because when something good is said after us, people do not hold it to last when something bad comes from us. This brings me to say that religious practice hinders a believer's relationship with God, and as a result of this, some believers do not know how a true believer should coordinate their affairs, therefore making it tricky at times to differentiate when a true believer is speaking and when a non-believer is speaking, apart from their actions which back it up.

However, it's our personal relationship with God that guarantees us staying in His commandments to reassure us that God is with us and reminds us through the help of the Holy Spirit to stay in His commandments so that we don't end up being disobedient children **(Proverbs 18:10)**.

(IV)

◯ Remember the Sabbath Day, to Keep It Holy ◉

Again, just as we should keep the name of the LORD divine, we are specifically reminded in this commandment to keep the Sabbath day sacred. The Lord blessed the Sabbath day, and it's the only commandment that carries a reminder, indicating a strong statement to illustrate that God knows that things would 'appear' more important but intended to remind the people to forget them to keep this law. Here is a reminder for people to maintain the Sabbath day as a holy day because it has been deliberately set aside and blessed by God, who has prepared this day with Him for us to be in His awesome presence. God expects us to set a time alone with Him, and our absence from God's table on this day defines dishonour to God.

Imagine that you have invited someone special for a date. You make special arrangements, and you order some unique things to surprise this special somebody. You don't want any distractions, so you arrange this date outside of town so that you can spend undivided and quality time with your invitee. However, you are aware that they do not have the means of funding the trip, so you arrange for private transport to pick them up from their doorstep to the venue and to take them back to their home. You don't stop at this length, assuring them that they will be fine while spending the day with you. You also reassure them by sending them a message to remind them about your arrangements and time. As a gesture of good will, you notify them to leave their purse behind so that they are fully assured that all expenses are on you.

However, on the day of the appointment, you turn up early and wait for them all day – but to no avail. They do not show up but give you a reason for not showing up, and although you accept this reason as genuine, after a repeat of this same performance for seven months, you come to the conclusion that they may not care as you care. Otherwise, you'd see some kind of commitment to match your energy.

What decision will you make next should this happen to you? Assuming that the special person is your teenage child or you are the teenage child, what will be your response to this scenario?

As such, the Sabbath day is the LORD'S day with His children. It is the day that the Lord has gifted to us as His children for him to unleash more blessings if only we can hear what the Spirit of the Lord is reminding us to do in honour of this day, which falls on a Saturday, by coming under His canopy to receive what He has prepared for us. An additional benefit for respecting this commandment is that our Lord has given us this day as a day to feed our spirit while relaxing our bodies, minds, and souls, with the assurance that as we hearken to this instruction, revelations and insights are breathed upon us as well as divine wisdom.

While we know that it is gainful to keep the Sabbath day holy, having gained divine wisdom, our deliberate, consistent efforts to honour this day for what it stands for will strengthen our relationship with God as we seek and search to see His mind for us. The people in this, like everyone in our household, are to enter into the Sabbath day with a different approach to the other days of the week because this is the day that the LORD has set aside; having created the world for six days, the almighty God Himself rested on the seventh day. Likewise, He wants the Sabbath day to be our day of rest, but He admonishes that we too will work for the remaining six days of the week.

Remember, this is the only commandment that comes with a reminder to treasure the Sabbath as a day of rest. Therefore, if we obey this commandment, we will ultimately see our mental health improved because it comes with a wellness package for the whole family.

> **'Blessed is the man who does this and the son of the man who lays hold in it; who keeps the Sabbath and keeps his hand from doing any evil.'**

> **— Isaiah 56:2**

(V)

◯ Honour Thy Father and Mother ◉

Children, you belong to the Lord, and you do the right thing when you obey your parents. The first commandment with a promise says, 'Obey your father and mother, and you will have a long and happy life.'

> **'Parents, don't be hard on your children. Raise them properly. Teach them and instruct them about the Lord.'**

> **— Ephesians 6:1–4**

We have just looked at how God has set the Sabbath day aside as a day of coming into His presence to grow a stronger bond with Him. We also saw that obeying the above commandment would enhance our well-being, and in so doing, God will reward us in return. Meanwhile, earthly parents are to mirror God's patterns and principal ways for guiding children into wellness. They are able to achieve this just by taking an example from the Ten Commandments to become like the character of God, which are in the structure of the fruits of the Holy Spirit (**Galatians 5:22–23**):

> **'But the fruit of the Spirit is love, joy, peace, forbearance, kindness, goodness, faithfulness, gentleness, and self-control. Against such things, there is no law.'**

What better way is there to lead our families forward than to base it on the law of love, which results in peace?

The enemy knows that disobeying God's commandments would bring destruction into the family environment and that this would create dysfunction within families. This is why the devil brings in a lot of distractions to divide us from our families. Some of these distractions come in through friends who may look like they mean well for us, but even if their initial intentions may not be bad, the enemy has a way of turning them into evil ones. In no time, if we allow ourselves to be around people who have little or no regard for their parents and families, we too may soon fall under the spell of disobedience and malice with our guardians/parents.

Just as God shows His children unfailing love and assurance, this is the way forward for parents and guidance to keep on showing this kind of love and forgiveness to their mortal children even if they cannot give 'agape' love because God is immortal. Love, as the Spirit of God gives us the grace to love, must be replicated in our family too to enable us win our family over to God if we maintain love and forgiveness. An example of this is seen when a rebellious child sees love and forgiveness demonstrated in the family continually. A picture of this type of forgiveness is seen in the story of the prodigal son and his father.

The prodigal son was possessed by the spirit of rebellion. As the story goes, one day the prodigal son told his rich father to hand over all of his inheritance so he could go fend for himself. Leaving his elder brother behind to labour in his father's yard, he left his family behind and went on a lavishing spree with his money. When his money was spent, famine swept over the land; this left him starving. He begged a local farmer to work in his animal farm so he could have some food. The prodigal son began eating with the pigs until he came to his senses and decided to go back home and beg his father for forgiveness, contemplating even working as a servant in his father's house. However, when his father saw him approaching the entrance of the compound, he could not wait to express his love for his son with an embrace at the entrance. The prodigal son showed remorse and repented and was reunited with his family.

In the first place, it was pride that made the prodigal son eat with the pigs because his pride made him forget who he was and where he came from, but he was driven by disobedience. In the journey of faith, disobedience reduces a man to nonsense. God hates these men who keep to their pride but enthrones the humble.

> **'But he giveth more grace. Wherefore he saith, "God resist the proud but giveth grace unto the humble."'**
>
> **—James 4:6**

God our heavenly Father is our spiritual icon for us to follow as an example of how to raise godly children to God's own standard and truth without compromising how the world preaches children should be raised. It is important to thoroughly understand the benefits of the commandments so that it will become easy to obey them.

'Honor your father and mother' is the only commandment that comes with a lifetime assurance of longevity and vitality; hence, it should be deliberately exercised if we want to retain the blessings that come with it. When parents and children are in line with all aspects of God's commandment, the family walks into the blessings of God rather than falling under the curses of God, which can be brought on by a single disobedience to God.

As the offspring of our earthly parents, we are meant to stay under the guidance of our parents and not insult them, even when we can make our own decisions as adults. We still give them reverence for their contributions in our lives and still have to accept their counsel because in it may be the wisdom that we need to deal with certain matters at one point or another in life. So that we can inherit the blessings that come from them and that they can teach us the way of life in a way that's fulfilling, we have to remain humble to them. Our destinies come at the appropriate time, but remaining in obedience with our parents has a way to stop abuse from coming to us and so allow us to avoid unnecessary delays to fulfilling such destinies, as seen with the prodigal son **(Luke 15:11–32).** Verse 21 highlights that the son came back home to beg for forgiveness and fulfil his destiny after he realised he had sinned against God for dishonouring his father:

> **'And the son said unto him, "Father, I have sinned against heaven and in thy sight and am no more worthy to be called thy son."'**

Disobedience to our parents brings dishonour into our homes. When we disobey our parents, we leave ourselves espoused in society to be subjects of stigma and shame. So we should try as much as possible to resist the spirit of rebellion and stay away from people who insult their parents because bad company corrupts good seeds, as clearly written in **1 Corinthians 15:33: 'Be not deceived: evil communication corrupts good manners.'**

Every child needs their parents' blessing, admittedly or not. When a son or daughter of any age is in dispute with their parents, they wear a bag of tension on their body, and this load is not settled until matters are resolved. In the worst case scenario, should the son or daughter lose their parents before they had the opportunity to make peace with each other, it is most likely that the son or daughter will live a large part of their life in guilt until they get fully healed. However, the healing session would involve a lot of work, both spiritually and physiologically, because while the mind is the strongest part of our being, the heart is, interestingly, the most vulnerable.

God blesses us to be blessings unto others; how much more would He release blessings to us through our parents? The cheapest way to bargain for this portion of blessings is to obey our parents, even though it is not the easiest way, because our parents are sometimes bound by their own belief systems that are ungodly and different from our faith.

The moral is that we have been created and chosen to be among the millions of survivors who exist in this world. While we did not make the decision to arrive in this world by ourselves, the almighty who created us already has a plan for us, both in the here and now and after life everlasting in this world. So our existence is not dependent on being here alone because there is also eternal life after exiting from this life, and this is also tied to this commandment: life after death. Also, God is committed to His part of the covenant if we continue to obey our part of the commandment.

There is blessing in obedience. This is how Abraham entered a sworn blessing from the Lord. God told the father Abraham that He will make him great across the earth, and everything that God told Abraham He will do for him came to pass, but first, Abraham was a bona fide obedient son and friend of God.

And I will make of thee a great nation,

And I will bless thee

And make thy name great,

And thou shall be a blessing,

And I will bless them that bless thee

And curse him that curseth thee,

And in thee shall all families of the earth be blessed.

Abraham's blessings for the nations of the earth came from God. Then Abraham passed on the blessings to his sons, Ishmael and Isaac. Isaac had two sons, Esau and Jacob. The scriptures record that when Isaac was old and about to die, he told his eldest son, Esau, to prepare him a meal so that he could give him his blessings before he died. Isaac wanted to pass on his blessings to Esau because of the close relationship they had. Unknown to Isaac, Isaac's wife, Rebekah, was listening to the conversation between Esau and her husband; because of the close relationship she had with her other son, Jacob, she told Jacob to go in disguise and collect the blessings from their father, who was old with dim sight and about to die **(Genesis 27)**.

(VI)

◯ **Thou Shall Not Kill** ◉

Do not kill anyone. This is what this commandment says – 'Don't murder' is 'Do not kill'. **Will the world be a better place if people stopped killing one another?** There will be less criminal activities if people do not murder one another, as this commandment says, but most people think that the commandments of God are foolish, and grievance is not knowing that they are to bless and enrich us if we obey them.

> **'This is the love of God that we keep his commandments: and his commandments are not grievous.'**
>
> **— 1 John 5:3**

> *'The day a person dies is not the day they are killed. A person dies alive when the soul of the person has been killed.'*
>
> **— Merisha Meisha**

(VII)

Thou Shall Not Commit Adultery

'Marriage is honorable in all and the bed undefiled: but whoremongers and adulterers, God will judge.'

— Hebrews 13:4

God will back up His word with His actions because He has sent His word ahead of time so that all men can benefit from it, whereby the raw hands of God cannot be stopped. This is why the scriptures still speak for us to study and listen to what the word is saying by doing what God has spoken.

The sin of adultery is considered very serious against God because God is the constitutional body of marriage between a man and a woman, so anyone who comes in between the husband and wife has come to put a division between God's covenant for the family because the marriage vow is taken in the presence of God, making God the source of their marital union. In as much as adultery is a sin of the flesh because it's committed with the body, adultery defiles the temple of God in one's body, which is meant to be kept consecrated. The nature of this sin pains the heart of God because its deceitful offence not only damages people emotionally, physically, and spiritually but also scatters both the immediate family and the extended family of those involved.

'You shall not commit adultery.' This is the seventh commandment that God has laid down among the ten commandments. Why would God put this commandment as number seven? The number seven is a very special number to God, as mentioned in the fourth commandment (how God rested on the seventh day). He chose the seventh day as a day to release His blessings to us. Equally, marriage is honourable because the Lord has poured out His blessings on marriages and sent His word to back them up.

Not everybody has to get married, although this is hard for many believers to embrace because they believe that to abscond from sexual immorality, marriage is the best option. While this may be the safest thing to do, this is not the best option to take, especially when the person or couple has not understood the key elements of marriage. The scriptures say that when a man finds a wife, he finds a good thing and obtains favour from the Lord. This means that it is more favourable to be married than to remain single. However, before sealing the courtship with marriage vows and commitments, the couple should study each other's characters very closely during the engagement period to see if they are compatible in different areas of their lives. They should also check to see if they agree on most crucial decisions they make regarding life issues that they might encounter on a daily basis regarding how they would run their family. First and foremost, they should see that they are of the same faith and believe in that system, as clearly questioned in **Amos 3:3: 'Can two walk together except they be agreed?'**

Henceforth, marriage is not the way out from adultery; in other words, having family problems in the household should not be an excuse for infidelity either. Rather, seeking marital counselling for reconciliation should be the way forward for every believer. However, where there's an incident of adultery, the Bible says that in this instance, a certificate of divorce is appropriate. Still, while divorce is appropriate in this instance, it does not mean that reconciliation cannot be considered; nor does it warrant a licence to hop out from a marriage agreement onto the next while the other partner is still alive. Hence, this is still adultery, and the consequence of disobedience is that which should be given equally to a sinner, as painted in this scripture:

> **'Know ye not that the unrighteous shall not inherit the kingdom of God? Be not deceived: neither fornicators nor idolaters nor adulterers nor effeminate nor abusers of themselves with mankind.' (1 Corinthians 6:9)**

Although this commandment is telling us not to commit adultery, God also frowns upon fornication. As seen already, adultery is a form of sexual immorality when a person in a marriage covenant has a romantic or sexual relationship with a person they are not married to. Fornication is another form of sexual immorality, but it involves a person who is not married having sex with someone else who is either married or not married. Most commonly, fornication is seen in the lives of young people who are of the mind-set that their bodies are theirs, so they can do whatever they like to do with them. Nevertheless, God is still angry even when His little children who are tender at age and immature in faith are being perverted by sexual immorality.

Whether known or unknown, the sin of fornication is a sin unto God because it is committed in the body of the person. The people of God are to keep their bodies holy unto God and use them in a way that God admonishes as they are created to be the temples of God, where the Holy Spirit resides.

Looking at the meanings of both immorality and sexual immorality, immorality is described as follows: 'the state or quality of being immoral; wickedness'. Meanwhile, sexual immorality is described as an evil act that violates social conventions: 'Sexual immorality is the major reason for last year's record number of abortions. Type of: evil, immorality, iniquity, wickedness' (*Vocabulary.com* www. vocabulary.com>dictionary).

You can see here that even the dictionary deems this act evil because of the consequence of this action, as described above. However, the severity of sexual immorality is downplayed in society, and unfortunately, most people of God have formed the habit of copying sexually immoral behaviour from society. Spiritual education on this aspect should be left open for enlightenment so that people of God can understand sooner than later that an aspect of sexual immorality is that after the enjoyment of sex comes downfall.

Most young people in the faith decide to get married early to avoid the sin of sexual immorality, but let's remember that while this is a good idea, it's better for any couple who have decided to get married to understand what the word of God is saying, particularly in the area that they have decided to venture into, so that they can treat and enjoy their marriage as a blessing rather than endure it as if marriage is living in bondage.

The best way to lead the children of God from the destruction of sexual immorality is to teach them about this topic and not shy away from it. Otherwise, they will learn about it through the ways of the world and inhabit the sinful ways of gaining sexual pleasure, which is easily accessible nowadays and includes pornography and masturbation. This can lead to sex addiction, which could make the person dysfunctional and potentially make them avoid a healthy relationship with the opposite sex in a blissful marital home.

Sometimes young people are discouraged from engaging in marriage discussions because when they hear other people talk about marriage, they mainly hear how marriage is terrible. This is because marriage is often described in the way the world looks at it, but the marriage that the word created is actually beautiful if only people know how to access it. The only time when marriage becomes painful is when people try to recreate it into what it's not designed to be in the first place and put their own opinions of what they want it to be; it gets confusing because one shoe does not fit all. That's why it's better to go back to the author and creator of marriages to ask for guidance on how marriage should be handled to build long-lasting marital homes that keep the marriage covenant.

'And the Lord God said, "It is not good that man should be alone. I will make him a helper comparable to him."'

— Genesis 2:18

A lot of the followers of the Messiah were asking Him about the laws of Moses regarding marriage. They enquired how it should be when a man wants to divorce his wife. A reply was given in **Romans 7:1–3**:

> **'Do you not know, brothers and sisters, for I am speaking to those who know the law, that the law has authority over someone only as long as that person lives? For example, by law, a married woman is bound to her husband as long as he is alive, but after her husband dies, she is released from that law and is not an adulteress if she marries another man. So if she has sexual [relations] with another man while her husband is still alive, she is called an adulteress. But if her husband dies, she is released from that law and is not an adulteress if she remarries another man.'**

I have spoken much more about the topic of sex in my book *Every Mind Matters to Messiah*, but coming back to the seventh commandment of 'Thou shall not commit adultery', here is what the word is saying in **1 Corinthians 6:15–20 (paraphrased)**:

> **'Know ye not that your bodies are the members of Christ? Shall I then take the members of Christ and make them the members of a harlot? God forbid. What? Know ye not that he which is joined to an harlot is one body? For two, saith he, shall be one flesh. But he that joined unto the Lord is one spirit. Flee from fornication. Every sin that a man doeth is without the body; but he that committeth fornication sinneth against his own body. What? Know ye not that your body is the temple of the Holy Ghost which is in you, which ye have of God, and ye are not your own? For ye are brought with a price: therefore, glorify God in your body and in your spirit, which are God's.'**

(VIII)

◯ Thou Shall Not Steal ◉

No matter how little a thing is, do not take whatever belongs to someone else because you don't know what it means to the owner.

What comes to your mind when you hear the word 'steal'?

For me, when I hear the word 'steal' mentioned, automatically, I assume something tangible, like a monetary or some materialistic item, but the most valuable items are not things. A person's confidence can be stolen if they are in an abusive relationship; for example, when this happens, most times, the person's spirit is crushed, leaving them in a somewhat low mood and ambivalence.

Other things that can be stolen from a person yet hard to prove are ideas. Surprisingly, this is common between a husband and his wife, especially if one is feeling inadequate in one way or another. For instance, this behaviour plays out when one of them steals the idea of the other as their own and then makes the other feel less valued in front of other family members. Unfortunately, the spouse who plays the role of the villain ends up stealing the voice of the victim. As if it were not bad enough that they stole the idea of the other in the first place, they mute them so as not to expose their spurious character.

Apart from someone's intellect being stolen, a person's reputation can be stolen if the person is being gossiped about at their place of work. The person is at risk of their image being tarnished and provokes people to discriminate against them.

'Time is the most precious [asset] in life that controls our movement but without any restrictions. God has our time, even though He has given us our freedom, so when our

*time is stolen, [this] is equivalent to our life
being taken and kept in someone's hands.'*

— Merisha Meisha

Time is one of the most irreplaceable assets in life, yet people's time can be stolen in different kinds of ways, both knowingly and unknowingly. For example, a person's time can be stolen if they enter a courtship with someone who is deliberately engaged in the relationship for selfish gains only. Ultimately, a person can also allow their time to be stolen if they know that they are being lied to by someone but remain in that relationship because they desperately want to remain in a relationship even if it's not fruitful.

*'Whatever [distracts] you from your given
task is stealing your time, and whatever has
come to steal your time [has] come to steal
your destiny, and whatever steals your destiny
[has] stolen your life.'*

— Merisha Meisha

(IX)

◯ Thou Shall Not Bear False Witness against Your Neighbour ◉

Lies are not just contagious; they also contaminate the heart of a person. As well, a liar always has his or her integrity at stake. It is true that lies start from the heart; however, their aim is to put a division between people, thereby setting confusion in their midst. The scriptures say, **'Every kingdom divided against itself is brought to desolation; and every city or house divided against itself shall not stand' (Mark 3:24).**

Lying defiles our character, and it is one of the sins wherein God said that for the people who do choose to lie, they will not see His kingdom. However, most believers think that the only way they can get past certain obstacles is by lying rather than seeing God as the rescuer from all obstacles who can provide exemption to all issues. Furthermore, a single lie has so many parts to it, while the truth stands as one and has only one part to it. Why then do we look at the sin of the body as serving, while lies are received as something 'only' trivial? Do we not know that God's anger is on people breaking this commandment, even as the Bible continues to reveal God's mind in various verses, such as those below?

> **'He that overcometh shall inherit all things; and I will be his God, and he shall be my son. But the fearful and unbelieving and the abominable and murderers and whoremongers and sorcerers and idolaters and all liars shall have their part in the lake which burneth with fire and brimstone: which is the second death.' (Revelation 21:7–8).**

(X)

Thou Shall Not Covet Thy Neighbour's Goods or Wife

The sinful nature of man is inherited from Adam and Eve, who are our very first parents on earth. However, we separate ourselves from the curse they carried on their heads after their disobedience, when they sought to find out the taste of the fruit from the tree of the knowledge of good and evil, which was against God's will for mankind as the tree was controlled by the devil.

In other words, we need to repent for our sins and evil ways to properly hear what the commandment is telling us to do. In doing so, we can choose to be on the Lord's side and walk in the way of His laws. This way, we are in constant communion with the word of God, which reconstructs our character and makes us better citizens in the community. By treating one another with love and respect, it is easy for us to place value on our neighbour, and in so doing, we cannot take advantage of their property or personality.

'No one can serve two masters; for either he will hate the one and love the other, or else he will be loyal to the one and despise the other.'

— Matthew 6:24

Acquiring the character of God helps us to behave like God. This means that we reform our old ways, and when we behave more like God, we are able to have self-control, discipline, and patience with one another. The lack of self-control leads to covetousness, and one of the online dictionaries describes covetousness as *'eager or excessive desire, especially for wealth or possessions that [belong] to someone else: "Social media so often encourages us to compare ourselves to others, inspiring covetousness"'*.

Often comparing ourselves with one another leads to unnecessary pressure, which increases the desire to become greedy for things that we cannot afford but want to acquire in our possessions. Many a time, these desires are what drive people to steal because they have not disciplined themselves with the word of God and depended on God for provision for their needs. Also, it is important to note that patience as well as self-control are among the nine characters of God, which are the fruits of the Holy Spirit **(Galatians 5:22)**. So when we make our requests known to God, we should also pray for the grace to be patient in waiting for the answers of our prayers to be delivered to us.

'Therefore, do not be like them. For your Father knows the things you have need of before you ask Him. In this manner, therefore, pray.'

— Matthew 6:8–9

If we have the conviction in our hearts that when we pray, God hears and grants us our requests, we would not be anxious for our daily needs. Rather, we should focus on advancing our spiritual needs, which would quickly reflect on our outer containers and increase our personal development.

As there is so much misconception among believers about prosperity, some believers think and behave as if they are better off remaining poor because they truly believe that Yeshua the Messiah was poor and, in turn, end up living lives of want and lacking, which lead to desire and depression. In the country, other believers think that they must be financially prosperous to express that God is with them; failing to incubate that wealth without spiritual enrichment is death as a believer's prosperity is for the kingdom's gain. God gives us prosperity in our finances so that we can provide resources for the less privileged in our community while preaching the gospel to them and, in turn, bring them nearer to Him and into His kingdom for them to be partakers of His wonderful works.

Using God's resources for what they are purposely designed for is paramount because whether believers realise it or not, non-believers are looking into the lives of believers. Apart from condemning them for the choices they make to follow God to the end of time, they are also detecting through the lives of the believers around them if it is appealing enough for them to be invited into the faith. However, if what they see is mostly appalling and not genuine, they will stay away, thereby at risk of falling under the disobedience of the ninth and tenth commandments, which are lying and stealing. As you can see, they both go hand in hand as both evils need skills to support the other to thrive in the victim.

There's a need to learn the skills of judging the temperaments of money matters so that money is not seen as evil or as a means to do evil unto others, whereby we take what is not given to us by force. Rather, money should be treated as one source of blessings so that we can be blessings unto other people in our community. God, on the other side, will send the right people to help us if we can just believe and not fill our minds with satanic wisdom and evil, plotting to steal from one another.

'But godliness with contentment is great gain. For we brought nothing into this world, and [it] is certain we can carry [nothing] out. And having food and raiment, let us be therewith content. But they that will be rich [fall] into temptation and snare and into many foolish and hurtful lusts, which drown men in destruction and perdition. For the love of money is the root of all evil: which while some coveted after, they have erred from the faith and pierced themselves through with many sorrows.'

— 1 Timothy 6:6–10

We must constantly strive to strike the balance of when enough of what we have is enough of what we need to avoid greedily seeking to purchase what our friends, family, or colleagues have at all costs, even if it means running into debt. Until our attitude to materialistic things in the world is reviewed with God's eyes through His word, we would not be more selfless people and care more for other people around us. Until we do this, our minds will not be more focused on the fulfilment of the Shekinah Glory, which will lead us to New Jerusalem, where the heavens come to the earth for us to have life's eternal enjoyment. Life's eternal enjoyment is for those who maintain their salvation and keep all commandments until the end of their days on earth; without having a constant influencer, we must have our minds made up to follow the way of God to the end of time.

'We must constantly strive to strike the balance of when enough of what we have is enough of what we need.'

— Merisha Meisha

In a changing world, the advancement of technology is making these changes faster. However, even with this increase, God's word is increasingly spreading across the globe so that everyone would hear the good news of the message our Saviour Emmanuel, the Messiah, King Yeshua Hamashiach, brought to His people so they too can be saved and inherit His kingdom.

'My son, give me your heart and let your eyes delight in my ways.'

— Proverbs 23:26

'For where your treasure is, there your heart will be also.'

— Matthew 6:21

Chapter III

 INSPIRATIONAL QUOTES BY MERISHA

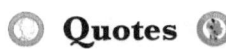 **Quotes**

Goal for growth: the truth is bitter, but if you bite it, you will be better.

Rule number one: praise God at dawn because you slept and woke up without knowing how.

Tomorrow there will be no more sorrow, so train your children today for their reign tomorrow.

Eaters are not takers, so eat to be satisfied and not full so you can stay on the runner's lane.

Talkers are not writers, so talk less and write on.

Don't talk your story through; write about it, and it will speak true for itself.

When your personality is beautiful, people would copy it, even those who hate you, but they can't steal your character.

Discipline, dedication, and determination would help you demonstrate your devotion for development.

By the time we run into the end of the road from where the enemy is pursing us, that's the beginning of the road where God starts with us to pursue a new beginning.

If you want an insider to follow you outside, sell yourself to an outsider.

It takes inspiration to think, but to produce, it takes creativity.

Life no be moimoi. If you no pray, Satan go play. In essence, life is not a joke; if you don't pray, the devil would have a wild time with your future.

Everything is done on TIME.

The TIME factor that control's a person's destiny allows the person to take full control of his or her own movements.

The accountability of how TIME is spent now would be demanded by God at the end of TIME.

TIME is to be mastered because the only thing that comes into your life in TIME is TIME, and the only thing that leaves your life with TIME is TIME.

The date of birth and date of death of a person are the two channels that bring a person into existence on earth and exit the earth through a concept known as TIME.

When the people you live with begin to check out from the house, one after another, take it as an indication that it's time for you to check in yourself.

Have a good sense of the TIME spent on your daily activities so that you are not in debt with TIME when it's TIME to account for your TIME spent.

At the end of TIME, it will be TIME for you and me to give accounts of how we have used the TIME that we were given.

Certain things happen to certain people in certain seasons for certain reasons to learn certain lessons.

When some believers stop worshiping people and focus their worship on God almighty alone, the majority of people worshiping idols would see a reason to focus their attention on God almighty alone in worship.

How you are treated among your friends is a reflection of how you respect your friends.

People would treat you how you treat your family. So the respect that you get from people is reciprocal to the respect that you give; you gain what is gainful for you if you do what is needful of you.

You give love to gain love. This is the law of the universe that cannot be cheated, not even by the entire universe.

Don't allow any worker to treat you like an institutional pay cheque.

If you can see the problem, you can see the solutions of the problem.

Science is based on facts, while the scriptures are based on truth. One changes; the other is everlasting. You decide.

One of the major problems people have is taking on other people's problems as their own problems.

Pride makes women not cover their hair when they come into the presence of the Most High, but the proud will He resist.

When I wear extensions and (make-up) foundation, I am telling God that He made a mistake in my creation, giving me an image that reflects His glory. I am also saying that the scripture that says I am fearfully and wonderfully made (Psalms 139:14) is a lie.

Good God; evil devil.

Don't give importance to an impotent devil whose desires are to infuse pain in the bone marrow of man so that he can stop men from having any relevance in the world.

An enemy is he who instigates fear in the system of his victim through any means or device whatsoever.

God is always proven right when He speaks by the sword of His word.

Dear God, please get me out of satanic dreams and cover my eyes with visions.

Yahweh, your ways always.

Let them gloat; give the glory to God and keep your glow.

Wherever there are winners, there are haters. Trust me – if you are on the winning side, you'll experience this. Keep winning anyway.

The next time someone asks me if I am a Nigerian, I will answer back with a question of whether it is a club or simply answer back with a small question of what makes a Nigerian.

What looks like fun when once done, when demons come, it will not be funny.

People be like 'You're crazy' when they see you in a war zone, but they have no idea what wars are hiding behind your walls. Keep fighting anyway; you're born to win.

Father, help me to believe in you more.

The sooner you understand the laws of forgiveness, the faster you will run.

Understand it now that to be gentle with your soul is to heal your mind, but to heal your mind, you have to forgive yourself first. Then your ability to forgive others will grow.

Never ask a baby why he or she is crying in a farmyard because you can't see the python that is smiling at that baby; only they can see it.

TIME is the breath of life. Spend it wisely, carefully calculating your journey with care in every single step.

Find the braveness, confidence, and courage to start doing a little kindness here and there, day in, day out.

Freedom is a kind of happiness which only courage brings when you allow yourself to be free from your oppressors.

One word from heaven is richer than a million promises from the government.

Have mercy on my soul, O Lord, and forbid my enemies to enter my future through my past.

Be kind to yourself; forgive in advance and enhance your love for yourself.

Many will gloat at your glory without knowing your story.

Yahweh will make a way always because He is Jehovah the creator.

Certain struggles are marks of the manifestation of unseen principalities fighting the destinies of people.

What laws you obey are dependent on what battles bow down.

Even if the addiction is strong, the mind is stronger.

When Yahweh's inspiration inspires you to speak of what is yet to come, it does not matter who believes you because when it comes to pass, they who concluded that it was fluke would see it happen, and even in their delusion, the conclusion will be blown in their flutes that God never lies nor fails.

Beat the odds and have a change of mind to look beyond the drugs.

TIME is focusing on what really matters. I have to ask myself how much I'm getting paid following this social trend. If the answer is zero, then I want to spend zero TIME looking at someone else's funny social media to build on more TIME developing my content to educate youths who will grow up to value their own TIME.

Anything that is worth doing is worth doing it on TIME.

When you gain the strength to forgive your offenders, you are halfway through the healing process of the abuse, but complete healing occurs when you gain the ability to maintain forgiveness continually.

Trust God with the process; if He brought you to it, He will take you out of it.

If you can see the full picture of what God is revealing to you at the beginning of the revelation, you will stay up pressing all night on it and can't wait to wake up to press forward with it.

Remorse is not repentance.

I'm so high on the all-Holy Ghost.

When you follow your dreams, you may end up in someone else's dream and slip, but when you follow your vision, you will read, run, and rise to the top.

Those who mock the word of God have refused to accept the works of God.

To all who laugh at me when I dance in the open air, if only you can see the stars in the blue sky; you'll be sure to dance with me.

Hold somebody's heart, tell them that you love their smile, be kind to them, and share a little laugher together.

Never fall in love. When you fall out of love, grow in love so you can stay in love with the person you grew to love.

Open the eyes of my heart, O Lord. I want to see you in my mind.

God, forbid me to be boastful in myself because with you, Lord, I am nothing.

A blind man whose eye is open for the first time wishes he could sleep with his eyes open.

I once met a deaf artist who said she is lucky not to hear all that people talk about in the world.

Open your mouth wide and tell Satan to get lost, and he will never return to you in the same area of temptation.

The faster you go without taking breaks, the slower you become; work smart and take care of your mental health.

Open the mouth of your mind and mediate.

We cannot all be on the same speed, or else, we will crash into one another at once in high speed.

Run your race and stay in your lane, for the race up the mountain is rough but beautiful at the finishing line.

If you are not yet at a stage where revelations with God become your normal way of conversation with God, keep going forward and refuse to look back until you begin to hear the voice of God swiftly.

The Messiah only said to the sea 'Be still' once, and the storm stood still at once. Everything stumbling in your life will tumble out of your life at once, and God will be praised because all the glory must return to Him. Amen.

COVID-19 made everything that was said to be abnormal appear normal, like singing in the garden, running in the garden, dancing in the garden, cooking in the garden, and drumming in the garden.

God changed my stories for His glory and gave me victory over theories.

The wicked cry when they hear saints sing.

Stop running to people who will feed you and start running to people whom you will feed.

I like upsetting the devil when I tell him I owe him nothing.

Once the intellect of a man's mind is deformed, you cannot transform him through his mind until his mind is reformed.

Polish the mind first. Then shine the light of understanding to activate the mind into tranquillity so that the information can be received and stored in the mind.

It is impossible to believe in what you don't belong to.

You can never fight a common enemy if you are with the one who throws the punches on your teammates.

Thank the heavens I never loved you more than I love God. Otherwise, I would not know how to love you like God loves me.

As a child of God, you are meant to help the poor, so you are not permitted to be poor. Otherwise, you will not be fulfilling the scriptures. Anyone who tells you otherwise is contending with your destiny.

Health is wealth, right? Get well in your mental health. There's no health without mental health as mental health is the engine behind physical health.

Come up a little higher to hear God more clearly.

I get the giggles when I read; when you find your happy place, stay there because it's your place of peace.

I empty myself every day so I can learn a new truth about myself daily.

I open myself up daily so I can reactive new wisdom from God daily.

Hearts are many, but love is rare. I stay with the stars and get no scars because the clouds are never rejecting.

Which of you is in a more prestigious place – you who is with the other and scared to go home or you who is alone and safe?

Seek peace and overtake it.

At my weakest point, I am so powerful because God's mercy locates me with more of His love.

Write a page a day, and you will end up writing a book in days.

Jealousy is a powerful substance that kills the villain yet makes the victim victorious.

Discipline is better than education if you know how to advance your skills because education is in practice and not in sitting.

You have to block some people if you don't want your blessings to be blocked.

Distractions are deposited in our direction for us to disconnect our walk with God. So they are dangerous demons directed to divert our destinations, thereby denying our destinies from developing at the set time.

I am not thinking about how I am writing, so my writing is rough. I am into what I am writing, so my writing is transparent.

To be a believer is a crazy phenomenon because you believe in things that are invisible and not yet in existence but come up with undeniable proof in TIME.

The day you collapse is not the day you die.

Your immune system dies before your body dies, but your body collapses first; then your immune system dies. This is when death takes over the person.

When you have a message from God for the people, run to the people, or else God will send someone else who can fly to reach the people before you.

When you have a message from God for the people of God, don't sit on it. Send it off at once because it will have an instant response, even if you can't see an immediate response; in the spirit realm, there would be a conviction that God is already in action, which will bring about a swift shift.

Your victory is either a fact mirroring your character or the maker of your character.

God's supremacy is sufficient enough for me because of His sovereignty.

God uses the available to make me capable.

If you want the rice, pay the price.

You know who your friends are when you're going down. Likewise, you know who is not your friend when you're going up, and when you're going up and down, you know who your real friends are.

Have the scriptures in you, not with you.

Once you have lost the use of your leg, you will never forget the use of your legs; walk while you can and run when you should.

The world's lockdown can never lock up your luck.

God's connectivity first will give you compatibility and enhance your communication.

I never thought I would live to see the day that the whole universe would be in lockdown at once, but this means, to me, locking in with God.

Check yourself to determine if your relationship with God is a deliberate, continuous, active action or by default.

Let my prayers not be a stain on my lips but the order of my day, O Lord.

Forbid me to forget to come into thy presence with pride.

Open my eyes so I can hear you more.

Sinners mock believers, but they are the real sufferers.

Let your authority determine your win, not the length of your lane.

Having the grace of GOD upon one's life is not equivalent to being safe in God's kingdom.

Don't get it twisted; worrying is not the same thing as caring. If they care enough, they will give you space and then knock on your door to see if you are OK.

Wait on God by trusting His timing as we follow Him and allow Him to lead us into the perfect day of Him delivering our requests to us.

Most of the time, we ignore the mind and focus on activities around the mind, forgetting that the outpouring of life comes from the contents of the mind.

When you gain the knowledge of fearing God, your behaviour reflects that fear of God, and your life becomes a witness of the fear and love of God.

Never allow yourself to be labelled as a statistic by the system and end up as industrialised personnel for a worker's pay cheque; thank God for the work of your hands and work on it.

The one who values you will respect your time.

It is better to give than to receive, but if you must love, you must give.

You can never be kicked and spat at by someone who loves you because love is gentle and accepting.

Through COVID-19, God is showing us different ways to worship Him, so we must worship Him in new ways.

Your talents are God's gift to you, but what you do with them is your gift back to God.

To seek God is to come closer and communicate via prayer. Listen and wait to hear a response, and even when you have not heard anything, study anyway while still waiting. As righteousness is becoming patient, begin to operate in wisdom from the knowledge gained while waiting. Begin to function in power of the wisdom, empowered on the go, and tell them to come and learn to seek Him first so that everything can be added.

Being afraid of being different is what robs you of your identity when the real fear should be looking like everybody else.

There is no one on earth fit enough to be compared with you; you are your own person, born bold and beautiful at a different time from everyone else, with a unique date of birth and a classic mandate.

If everybody likes you, it is because they can tell you are going nowhere higher than them.

When you serve God with your TIME, He will multiply your talents in no time.

Use your talents to draw men nearer to God, and He will make you a blessing to all men.

Remember, it is not how many followers you have but how many people whose lives you have impacted that matters.

If you can impact one person, then you have impacted a million persons.

Do not allow your beauty to fade away by feeding your body substances that are not a natural for your body.

Remember that what goes into your body affects your mind, what affects your mind affects your life, and what affects your life interferes with your living.

The decisions you make today affect the dimensions you accomplish tomorrow.

Handing out money to a person is not the help they need to bring them higher. Real help is demonstrated by holding the person's hand in yours and then the both of you walking together on a platform that would lift them up and out of a pitiful phase in their life.

Laughing at someone does not make them better about themselves; it just reveals how deeply those words pierce into their mind.

The world is a creating space, created out of creativity by the creator who created us to create, so get up and be creative.

For most things that were not seen as normal, the COVID-19 pandemic has made them seem normal.

No genuine Bible student seeking the knowledge of God has a graduation date from the school of thought.

God's mind for people is of love for the world and humanity for mankind.

Forgiving others is the key to healing oneself because bitterness eats up the bones.

To be an adult is to take responsibility for one's actions no matter the participants. Always own up to your contribution in a matter.

Look for resolutions to enhance progression to avoid regression.

'Seek before you receive' is the reality when looking for the face of God on a particular matter because when you knock on the door, you expect someone to ask, 'Who is there?' However, that someone behind the door also expects you to answer, 'It is I,' following your name. We should apply the same principle when we go to God, asking for help in our prayers, because our prayers are our communication links to God. So don't be in a hurry to get going until you have heard Yahweh say, 'It is "I am that I am" you are looking for. I have heard you. Now this is the direction you should follow.'

The whole point of fasting is to permit yourself to go beyond your limitations so that you can allow God to take you above your limits.

Never allow the seed of jealousy in your eyes to germinate into the tree of hate in your mind and produce the fruits of bitterness. This will grow into a tree of bitter fruits in the body which can develop into cancer if the tree is not uprooted aggressively with the blood of Jesus.

One's intellectual status is not to be boastful about. This is pride, and the scriptures say the proud bring disgrace, but with the humble is wisdom, and the meek will He honour.

Disobedience of God's leading leads to the destruction of one's life.

Distractions are dangerous devices which the devil uses to deter our direction so that he can make us deviate from our destined place of occupancy.

When we are challenged, the devil creeps into our minds with lies to victimise us so that we will not have harmonious lives, but God comes with His promises to enable us to live with joy so that we can be victorious.

'It is wrong to serve the almighty living God.' I will serve Him anyway. Even if it is wrong to serve God, I will serve Him anyway, and if it is right to serve God, still will I serve Him with an abundance of joy.

Decide whom you believe; then follow their ways. God is heavenly, but the devil is hellish. Choose one way. As for me, I say whether it is right or wrong to praise God the almighty living Father, creator of the universe, still will my praise go up to Him all the way.

When you deny the devil the chance to steal your laughter, he can never steal your star. When your star is shining, your joy can never be taken from you; with your joy lit up, you can light up the lives of others who are in a dark place.

When your mind takes you for a race, remember to take it for a walk; take it on a stroll and rest its pace.

To use a positive action to correct a negative reaction, there must be zero criticism applied.

If you always leave the other person crushed after every argument or disagreement, check yourself and remove the dark spot on your chest before it becomes a stain on your mind, which will, in turn, poison your heart.

It takes every hour for the burglar to collect a few items periodically, but it only takes one minute for the occupant to recover all at once.

Give one another space and ensure firm boundaries to prevent matters from escalating.

Choose to be victorious and not a victim because victims of a subject attract flies, and flies perch on wounds and shit out worms that turn into shit.

Stagnant water stinks. Keep flowing until you overflow and begin to fill other people's buckets.

Permit your praise to be louder than your prayers this day.

Build yourself up to be the one who can not only give feedback but receive criticism, yet reject them who only come to criticise.

Whenever you read the scriptures, be sure to study them so that you can hear what the Lord is saying in the 'here and now' for you to apply it into your own life.

It is impossible to exclude God from the knowledge of His creation because God's sovereignty is the source of His supernatural wisdom.

Reorganise your heart first before organising your house because your heart is where you welcome others to you.

The way to the Lord is to give Him your heart, and He will show you His mind.

Formerly, when I heard people say 'demon', I thought it a force that propels a person to carry out an evil act against another person. I never thought of it as the evil that occupies a person and accrues evil activities inside the person.

Demons are the devil's naked multiples in disguise inside a clothed personality.

Even the devil likes to steal pure and purified things. What a filthy demon!

Run to God to the extent where the demons pursing you will begin to follow your God.

Angels are the quiet ones who help God bring a person into noiseless breakthroughs, while demons are the utmost noise-making devils that aid Satan in bringing a person into detriment.

Peace can only be claimed when the wind can be calmed right in the midst of the storm.

Sometimes God puts you in a place alone so that you can realise that all you need is Him alone for all your needs, including your natural and supernatural needs.

Hide yourself so that the next time your enemies think they can meet you in the same spot you found them, they will be disappointed to see you at a top spot where they have never contemplated climbing and never comprehended reaching to catch up with you.

'Beautiful' is no longer pretty if it is available to everybody.

Thank you, Lord, for the test. Lord, I thank you for enabling me to sit still while waiting for you to help me pass me through this pathway of trails triumphant.

I thank you, Baba God, for giving me the grace to complete this race without grazing my knees on the grass.

Father, I thank you for empowering me to receive your grace, to be empowered, to receive your anointing, and for anointing me to receive your power.

Utmost muteness is not quite quietness when the mind is palpitating.

If you've not learned how to be happy alone with yourself, you will find yourself lonely in a group of happy people.

You don't win in prayers sitting down because a war is never won sleeping.

Salvation is the gospel proclamation of the good news of Christ and the receiving of Christ to service one's life to be right with Christ.

I am a believer of words; I am no fool, but I am full with love.

Defeating demons demolishes deaths.

Clever people hide inside the closet while creating; their work brings them outside, on a public stage, for display after creating.

A child becomes an adult when they lose their parents at a tender age, but a cat becomes a lion when it returns from a trip alone – a lone trip talking with God.

Don't decide to kill yourself today because someone turned off your lights yesterday. God can decide to show you where the switch is after you have dried the tears from your eyes.

Don't kill yourself today if you can't find your fish in the basket. Tomorrow may deliver twelve full baskets of fishes for you to celebrate and have plenty left over.

Those who make televisions do not sit in front of the television. They remain the engine behind the scenes so that they can be visible on the screen.

World changers do not steer the world, moving round the globe; they move around globally, changing the world.

Give yourself a realistic due date when setting goals so that you can score your goals while on the go.

Delight your heart with all diligence and practice what you preach at all times.

Walking into God's calling and following His lead is like hearing the voice of God saying, 'Come to me, my child. Stay with me, my child. Now go for me, my child.'

The spirit controls everything; life is a spirit, and there is a spirit working behind every behavioural emotion.

You learn a lot about how others feel about you when you get in touch with how you feel about others and learn about your relationship with yourself and how you feel about yourself.

You learn a lot about how other people feel about things when you get in touch with yourself and how you feel about things.

Dyslexia engages my mind with a creative fuse.

Thank you, Lord, for making me stay in my mind and not in my head. This way, I can be certain to hear from you and not from me.

To acknowledge good behaviour, we have to give praise and rewards, but to encourage good behaviour, we have to apply discipline.

Be incredibly wired! Stand out.

Use little strokes to create giant waves.

Keep calm. The Holy Ghost is at work.

Even if it looks like nothing is working in front of my door, I know my angels are working hard behind closed doors.

If only each challenge knew that it would form part of the bricks that have built me up, it would have had second thoughts before coming to break me down.

God picks up the broken pieces of a table mirror and remodels it into a standing mirror.

Get rid of your destructive self and allow room for your constructive self.

If the story has nothing to do with me, then I don't know anything about it.

God's art of love is in His act to the people in His ark of peace.

It's difficult to think about it and not be able to talk about it, but it's more difficult to think about it and not be able to write about it.

The best way to learn is to empty your mind of everything you have already learned about the subject so that you can refill your mind with everything you will learn about the subject.

Even when you don't know how to do it, when God says, 'Do it,' just do it.

Anyone can write a book about anything, but not everyone will write a book about anything.

God says 'Do it.' I don't know how, but I will obey, and angels will accompany me as I accomplish the task.

When God sends you to do a task, He sends His angels to accomplish the task with you when you move.

When you move, God moves with you, just like that.

It is wickedness for a person to strip from another everything about them that they fell in love with in the first place.

Most times, what you are fighting is not what is fighting you. Some invisible battles are the result of what you have underestimated as trivial because it remains unseen.

This day, I promise to keep my head up! I will start this week with jam-packed positivity, creativity, and productivity.

Focus on the right things. In the meantime, God's time is really the best, so wait for His prompting and remain in His lead.

Once upon a time, I was so lonely, I forgot I had a self, but today I recognise myself and am happy to be alone but not feel lonely.

Some give themselves to others, waiting to be accepted when they themselves have not yet accepted their own person.

I have observed people from all over the world talking about mental health as if it's a thing that they can pluck from a tree with a stroke and that will fall off the skull of a human being. Others react as if mental health is something that they can catch from the air and throw into the rivers to flow to far countries.

Saying my mental health matters encourages me to talk about my own mental health as openly as I talk about my physical health. Physical health is not superior to mental health, but there's no health without mental health.

You don't win a fight sitting down and cannot win a war sleeping.

In every minute, there is a second chance for you to seize an opportunity and help someone you don't know.

When you offer your shoulders to just one person, you will never run out of people offering you their shoulders.

Be the sunshine on a foggy, misty day.

If you see every day as a passing season that can never be backdated to the present time, you will make the most of every ticking second in time.

He downloaded our daily benefits into us, which means there is wisdom added to us daily. Ask for it.

Sometimes when I see my quotes, I smile and think, 'What was I thinking of when I thought of that?'

If you want to see changes in the world, you must change what you are doing in your world.

Don't become a snob to contentment for spectacular moments because when the lights go dim, the spark would fade away faster, but contentment keeps the spark on the candle as the night fades into the morning.

Never despise your past. You don't know what that experience has prepared you for your tomorrow; even though you cannot see it today, keep on pressing ahead for a better tomorrow.

Plan to progress and stay in the process; press on, and you will soon discover where to pass.

Give power to the people who are working for the people.

Failing to plan is equivalent to planning to fail.

Falling is not failing. Failing is falling and failing to get up when you are falling.

When something new happens, something different has to happen.

God will never force anyone to obey Him, but a drastic situation may force somebody into obedience to God.

A wealthy man determines his family's banking system.

God can use an ant to disgrace an antelope just to establish His grace.

The girl whom God uses is not perfect but perfectly made whole in her obedience to God's leading.

Die every day for others to live well daily.

God still speaks if you tune into His frequency.

God has not given us the spirit of fear, so if you are operating in fear, you need to bounce into faith and keep still. Our angels have been sent out to work on our behalf, and the Holy Spirit of God is working things out even if you cannot see it.

Reading the word of God reveals God to you through the revelation released.

What matters to Martha meant to Mary that Martha was not mastering matters about Mary's matters mattering to Martha.

The only food I have for you is the word of God so you can go and feed your street kindly.

Realise the vision and activate your mind to the mission.

Honour is pregnant with favour, yet transgression gives birth to frustration.

If there was too much noise in the room of the artist, there would be no space for creativity in the artist's mind.

I am not on Facebook because I need to face my book.

If we cannot get over it and cannot get under it, then we must get through it.

Thank you, Lord, for bringing me this far so far. I trust that you have brought me to it, I see you are taking me through it, and I thank you for letting me go over it so that I can come out of it because I cannot get over it until I have gone through it, and if I have not gotten over it, I will be under it.

The devil is not afraid of you, but he's scared of what you know about your faith in God. This is the main reason he comes as a thief to steal the joy of the saints so that he can hold them down in fear.

The enemy comes with confusion to suppress and depress, but the saviour comes with liberation and freedom to set the captives free.

Satan says 'Close your mouth' so that no one would hear you screaming for help or shouting in joy, but God says, 'Open your mouth, and I will fill it up.'

Adding generosity to the good that you do multiplies the goodness in your deeds.

If a mouse comes out from a hole and tells you that there is a snake under the ground, believe it because household wickedness is real, and the enemy is always near, but God is even nearer.

When distractions slip into my mind, I sometimes become mentally disoriented. It brings my movement into a halt, like a spine controlling my brain linked to my legs, which makes my time spent on an activity stand still until the next day, like a total eclipse. I notice, yet I press on to complete my work.

All blessings come from God through men to men.

Honour is what lifts you up from the grass to grace and turns your life from reproach to rejoice.

Be a detective of your destiny and detect the songs of distraction so as to be quick to walk away from it. When the devil fails to distract you, he will use someone you are sensitive about to descend upon you and remove your attention from your focus so that he can steal your crown and glory. Still, you must remain focused and keep pressing on until the end of the project at hand.

Things will work out. Just trust God always and remain humble, pluck up some courage, and wear a smile, especially in difficult times.

There is a pandemic of drugs among youths all over the world, but the dealers must tell them that they will mess up their young minds from every angle, as they did with theirs.

Walk faster to work smarter.

Every time you reread your book, you rewrite your book as if you are writing it for the first time.

The best books are written from your head without any external resources. Everything you need is already available to you from the day you were born and stored in your mind until the day you are ready to release it from your hands.

People do not buy your person; they buy your discipline. You must separate yourself from other people to become the person whom they can buy, for it takes discipline to discipline yourself.

If you can't tell your testimonies in the space of a minute, write a book of testimonials and dedicate it as a memorial to God for His goodness and mercies in your life.

If you can believe in an invisible killer as COVID-19, surely, you can believe in an invisible healer such as the HOLY GHOST.

You can't receive anything with your hands wide open until you open your heart wide to retain it.

Humility is the gateway for victory.

Generosity is the key to greatness.

Dedication, discipline, and determination – time works better when you have these three in order.

Dedicate your time to something, be disciplined to commit to it, and be determined to see it completed.

God is ahead of TIME, but he has announced the season for greatness to be now.

Lost patience kills your faith; hold onto hope to keep faith alive.

When you are climbing up, the only people who can stop you is a person, and that person is you.

If your lights are in the dark, they will restrict your vision. You cannot tap currency from someone who is drowning you with his or her sorrows. A blind man leading another blind man would lead to them both slipping into a deep pool.

Stability, stamina, strength are all the source of success.

If you don't want to hear my test, how can you enjoy my testimony?

A man without God is blank.

God can use anybody to roll away your obstacles, but if there is no one available, God can use an ant to roll away a stone on your path to see that you don't trip over the stone.

Believers believe.

The People's People: My Mental Health Matter Ministries work through the word of faith and dance in praise because God is a people's personality, and He created people to praise Him.

The enemy's weapon to break your arm and hold you down in fear is guilt, but you disarm the enemy with your weapon of faith and rise to freedom through grace.

Die every day to live daily.

God is still speaking if you listen carefully.

It takes faith to kick fear out.

Stop going around looking for miracles; keep still and be the mystery of the miracle to be delivered.

The devil knows what you will gain from reading the book *Satan, Get Lost*. This is why he has kept into your business and kept you busy, busily looking for businesses, because he does not want you to know your own business so that you can be busy with your business.

Realise the vision, activate your mind, and map out the depression.

Anything against your happiness is against your life, so you must learn to cut it off before it cuts you off.

Trim off jealousy before it strips you of your strength.

If there's too much noise in the room of an artist, there would be too little space for the artist to create, but the louder the noise upstairs, the neater the creation.

The absence of faith permits fear to steal your rights.

A fellow student once criticised me for being overly prepared before a group process session. I cried. Then I was criticised for crying, so I became afraid of crying and kept mute. Then I was criticised for the lack of participation. Then I became expressive, and I was chosen as a student ambassador to represent the whole student body. Not every criticism is designed to break you; some are designed to build you up, but you must not conform with the criticism as your true self because what they see is not what you are becoming.

First, sit down and write about it. Then stand up and talk about it.

The eyes of an artist are like those of an eagle but with a frenzied mind of aesthetic pictures.

Get yourself alone with God in the early mornings, and He will stay with you until the late hours.

A little girl is given all she needs until her wants become her needs.

As first-time parents, we seem to derive the needs of our little person from our wants but misinterpret them as basic needs for them.

You win the race of life with stamina, not speed.

God works in any way to make His way work.

You maintain good communication with God when you consciously open up your spirit to sink in with the Spirit of God. However, in aligning your heart with this activity, be mindful to work from a concentrated mind so that you are working towards the delivery of the message you've received from the Spirit to the people you've received it for.

If you want the kind of love you desire, you have to give the kind of love you need.

Talking pages in my head – conversations with the Holy Ghost are without confusion but filled with insightful, blissful illumination.

One among the many things that I have learned from the power of reflection is that a person is determined to kill himself or herself because the pain they feel is too much.

The world keeps implementing systems to frustrate God's followers, but God keeps creating avenues to make Christians soar like eagles.

It is the enemy that injects hates into our minds, but together, we fight against one another through our own stubbornness and wound our souls with the sword of pride yet refuse to heal one another with words of forgiveness. Now that we are no longer foolish, we can perpetuate the love.

An artist needs a silent space in their mind to draw a loud picture on the surface.

Until outsiders begin to buy your work, insiders will never appreciate your worth.

I am addicted to reading the word of God because I hear them aloud in revelation and see proof in their testimonies.

Work in silence and allow your testimonies to scream in volumes.

Thank you, Lord, for your revelations remind me of your promises.

If your thoughts are good, they will beam out of your face like sunbeams, and you will always be caught smiling for no apparent reason, but just in your thoughts, you're alive.

Find happiness in yourself first; then take this happiness out to others next.

Make that 'someday' be the day that you can say, 'I can, I should, and I will do it.'

You can never be single if you have a relationship with God; let it fit your mind-set.

Toxic people – love them from a distance so that they don't contaminate your love for the rest of the world.

An enemy is someone who hates to see you smile.

The devil is within; when you can defeat him in your 'mind-field', you will win against him in the main field.

The battles of life are won in the invisible fight that takes place before it manifests into the visible fight, but victory is claimed in the open.

Never stop being the best you can be, even when you are not appreciated; those mistreating you are reflections of who they are, not what you are.

If you can't be nice when I show you my scars, be silent when I peel off the plasters because it took faith for me to see them clip the stitches on my skin.

It is the family that is mad, not the individual, and if the family is mad, it is the nation that is mad, not the family, and if the nation can be mad, then the world must be a mad place, not the people, so never call a person who looks and acts different from you mad because you never positioned yourself to advance their sanity. Mental health matters where it matters most.

Stop asking people for affirmation because they would always prescribe you to their descriptions, and you'll never find your true nature.

The scriptures say, 'Fear not.' Do not fear.

Anything pursuing your peace is after your life – RUN!

All vanity will vanish when vivacity kicks in.

Thank God my mother never aborted me, or else I will not be here today.

Every single parent knows this: God has blessed you with your children. Therefore, as you do His works by raising those children, He has already blessed the work of your hands and will multiply your blessings, just like He blessed Hagar and gave her a son, Ismael, and out of him came a nation.

As I praise you, O Lord, take me on a ride on your wings, hide me under your shadows, and make my bed with your feather in the clouds.

Everybody has something in them that they can offer to someone else to help them solve a problem.

All parents know this: your children came from the Lord, so raise them to His standard without any compromise. Love them like how you claim God's love in your life and lead them to become what He created them to be, not what you think would be beneficial financially.

You can never appreciate joy if you have never understood pain.

I see the pages of the scriptures painting pictures of my future.

Be mindful of how you treat those who cross your path because you don't know how your footprints would leave permanent marks on their minds.

Show the credibility of what you can produce before you go for funding; develop your content, and it will be easier for you to demonstrate your commitment.

God prepares us for our roles before He enthrones us.

Grow your mind so as not to see gossip so that your soul will not feel the offences and so that your heart can continue to replicate love for all.

Increase your hope so that your health can be enhanced.

The end of hope is the beginning of the end of good health.

The wicked are weak, so they prey on those who are steady and fast on their feet to make them weaker because they can see that they are strong in faith.

It does not matter who does not believe you as long as you believe in what God has told you.

He who has told you He will will perform as He has told you, for He is committed to perform in what He says. All you have to do is keep believing in His promises no matter who does not believe in Him.

When low self-esteem comes to deny me who I really am in God, I look in the mirror and announce that I am perfect in God, who made me whole already.

Sometimes when I am so afraid, I tap into boldness and see faith working like fire, and the fire overthrows the fear that almost consumed me.

The highest form of prayer is to give praise to God because your praise validates your prayers and demonstrates faith in God.

Lord, shine your light on me and bring my light to break forth so I can see a new road and direction ahead of me in the mighty name of Jesus.

Whatever is worth doing is worth doing quickly.

Increase your prayer time, increase your word time, and increase your praise time, and God will increase His presence in your life.

What eyes and ears have not seen and heard must be my experience this year because I have taken the responsibility of exercising my walk with God in a new way.

It is by God's grace that I am alive today, so I must subscribe to His grace daily.

God's word is my empowerment and lifts me; hence, it takes me out from depression and gives me the strength to keep pressing towards my vision.

God's purpose for my life is for me to prosper and fulfil every vision that He has shown me.

Prophecy for the future chases away fear of the future.

Whatever you commit your heart to do, God compliments your hands to complete it.

Choose to rejoice and confuse the devil so that whenever he comes with pain, you grab your gain and run with joy.

God chooses a person out of a group of people because He saves a person to rescue the people he wants to save.

Gather us together for your greatness in the world, O Lord, so that we can spread goodness to the rest of the world, thereby making the globe a place where your generosity can be replicated.

I heard my father say one day, 'You cannot be bored with all the books in the house.' I say you can't be bored with the vision boldly written in front of the television.

Forgive me, Lord, if I have fixed my eyes on people and things; Holy Spirit, I welcome you in my life today, and I place my hope on you alone.

My assignment is to go into the world and preach the gospel to the world, starting from my home town and city. So help me God.

God is not an 'I' God but a 'people's personality' God.

Lies stink; they fly and sting.

God has no problem with your past; rather, He is more interested in your future. Return to Him, and you will see Him resume his work as He was never absent.

I am a blessing to every man and a flavour to the world.

Wonderful Jehovah, show me which switch I need to turn on daily to keep the peace in my home. Then give me the wisdom I need to lead my home each day.

A few days is a thousand years in the absence of patience.

In the school of knowledge, there are no ceremonies for graduation – expect for a change of classes.

The works of our Lord Jesus for my life were finished on the cross, but His works in my life will not be finished until the perfect day when I meet with Him.

Every delay in your life has been crushed, all delays have been terminated, and the favour of God has lit up your soul today in the mighty name of Jesus. Amen.

You must continue to speak it forth to see its force.

Every revelation from God should deliver a revolution to the world.

God is showing you new stages because He wants to make you a show on these new stages.

If you don't like how you're being treated by someone, keep changing how you react to their treatment. You cannot control how they treat you, but you can control how you respond to them as you are responsible for your actions, which are controlled by you.

What you prepare for will only happen once you are prepared to break the bridge of your stagnation and walk into your breakthrough.

Most temptations germinate from seeds that were sown in the mind; if you uproot the seed, then you can overcome the temptation.

Time can never be rewound; play with sand like cupcakes and with dollhouses while in childhood, for when you grow into adulthood, sand will be for building houses, and dolls will be given to your children to play with in the dollhouse.

You need to catch the bird before it flies away, just like how you need to be quick at jotting down inspiration as soon as it lands from heaven; be consistent in taking note of it because just like the wind, once it blows, it goes and never blows back the same way.

My greatness can never be hidden because I am a city lit up on top of a mountain.

Nobody can ever make anybody happy because happiness is what you bring to the table and not what you take from the table.

Dear Lord, make my belly a carrier of joy.

Forgiveness is a powerful tool that you can use to set yourself free from the enemies' den.

If you charge yourself one coin for each time you waste a second, you will be in debt with yourself.

The gospel of my God – who is the everlasting, almighty living Father – is progressive; while it has the same components of the old, I believe we are made new through Jesus, our Lord and personal saviour.

The devil displays different distractions at different times; some distractions are to discompose, to cause dysfunction, and others are set out to destroy destinies. Some dismiss the presence of God from the lives of people, while many others bring death. To escape these distractions, we need to master the skills to deviate from the devil's distractions by diverting the devil from our roots when we keep quiet about where we are going, thereby directing the devil to fall back into his corny plans of destruction.

You don't need to have money first before you can think of your options. Think of your options first; then you will have a reason to increase your avenue on how to source the money to fund your options.

Every instruction from God is for our construction.

If you cannot see it, you cannot reach it, so change your mind set and set your eyes on the vision so that your hands can catch it.

What you say is what you get. Praying without activating your mind is like pouring water into a basket.

Snake's hiss, Judas kiss – beware of every **frenemy** because you don't taste the bitterness until the kiss is over, but when you hear the hiss, it is the right time to run, so don't wait for the kiss before the chase.

God is not limited, so let's not entrap Him in the building of the church alone with parochialism because God wants solidarity in society.

I can't contain God in a container, for His outstretched arms go all round the entire universe, just like His eyes roll round the world at once because of His sovereignty.

The people of God are a moving people. The word of God said the gates of hell cannot prevail when God builds His church. So empty yourself and allow your spirit to move with the Holy Spirit.

Success will not fall from the top; everything meaningful and worthy of your time has got to be built up, from bottom to top.

Satan can come in so many different ways; look around you with your mind's eye, and keep the windows of your house wide open. Keep your gob closed but remain in prayer so you can direct any angel to fling him out.

Lies are an illness. One can only get well from it if they treat it as a sickness that needs healing. Then healing will only occur after the realisation that lies are actually sins.

When the devil wants to break into a home, he will first open the door with confusion, but when the residents of the house make God their landlord, they can use God's master keys to lock the devil out because God is the author of peace and not confusion.

I did not know I could perfect it with faith until I walked in perfect faith.

I would rather lie in wait than to settle with a liar because a liar can steal and deny things, but a thief could steal and admit that he or she stole something to satisfy their hunger.

Murder is not far from the hands of a liar.

Do not judge a person whom God is using by his or her outer appearance. God sees the purification of their heart and the readiness of their mind.

While men see the imperfect and condemn them, God sees the condemned and perfects them.

If I had not known God's love, I would have fallen for lust again and lost my life waiting to be loved because anything that wastes your time is causing you to waste your life away, so you must kill it fast.

Thank you, LORD, for loving me first. I can never love you more, but I live my life to love you always.

One lie wipes off a thousand truths.

If I have impacted one person, I have impacted a million people.

Happiness is not when you are with someone and happy but when you are happy with yourself. Happiness is who you are within yourself, so you have to be happy with yourself first before you can be happy with others.

Faith lifts up our souls to hope for joy to fill our hearts with love.

The love that makes you fall will not be the love that lifts you up; be lifted with love because love is uplifting.

I fall in love with Jesus first, and now through His spirit, He has shown me how to stay in love so that I don't fall in love but grow in love.

My walk of life is about me discovering my journey and then God releasing me to the world as a destiny helper.

If God has shown you your vision, write it down fast and work on it quick, or someone else will sell it to you with a discount but charge you twice for it.

Don't clutter my mind with junk. I have just cleared out the clutter and made room for creativity so there's no room for junk.

Creativity without productivity is like breathing without taking in oxygen.

The devil will use the sin that is familiar with your habits to make you sink more into sin.

Avoid aggressive moments; be progressive and do not allow the weeds of bitterness to block off your pathway.

Anything you have accomplished becomes easier to replicate.

I did not pen down the inspiration then, but it flew and perched on my mind, just like a bird that pokes into my cap.

When the going gets tough, the tough gets going; the pain kicks in worse than ever just before the healing takes over, so never give up hope.

Just when they say you can't walk with your legs, get up and use the arms of your mind to walk.

Once you have been locked in with God, the effect that you have been with God must be evident.

The grace of God is mightier than the might of men and greater than self-reliance.

God called me first to come to Him. Next, He ushered me to stay with Him, and then He sent me out to go for Him.

A man who does not understand the factor of TIME is like a man sitting on a TIME bomb.

Disobedience to God brings on disgrace to the self.

I am faster when I am fasting.

Worrying does not warrant carrying; don't get it twisted.

God can use an ant to humiliate an antelope just to disgrace the peacock that fails to realise that being without the grace of God is not better than grass on the ground.

We have to make decisions on what we want to become first before the decisions we make can turn us into who we need to become.

Without discipline, motivation comes to nothing. You need discipline to empower what motivation thinks is possible, but discipline is what makes that thought a reality. Motivation gets you out of bed; discipline keeps you in your seat.

Those who change the world don't travel round the world collecting souvenirs; they tour round the world with their minds making changes for the world through the creation of their hands and then teach the world to implement those changes.

Looking back to move on should be just a glance back, or you may end up in a ditch.

Once you see the light switch up in the mountain that switches on the light so that you can see which direction to take, the next time you go up the mountain, you will not walk around in darkness because you will know where to switch on the light. Whenever the devil tries to blind you, keep him in his own blind spot, and he will never try to hold you captive again in the same area you walked out of darkness from.

It is your attitude towards gratitude that enhances your aptitude to create; keep on tanking God for your creation, and He will multiply your creativity.

Going back into darkness after seeing the light is like choosing cheap wine over fine wine.

The devil uses useless ideas to cause confusion because he is full of darkness, evil, and satanic wisdom.

You need courage to take the first step up the stairs God wants you to climb, and then faith will lift you up to the top of the stairs. You need courage to take faith; be encouraged.

Don't worry about who makes fun of you when you are working on your vision; it is because they can't see the pictures that God is showing you.

Don't mind who does not understand you now. They will see more of you later; then they will understand you better.

I am drunk daily with my vision, and this keeps me happy, doing what God is showing me to do.

Climb up to the bridge of joy to get to the mountain where thy Lord has prepared your palace.

My life must not be cut short. I must live a life that is full of light. My life must end well, and other people must benefit from the brightness of my light.

Don't behave and act from the realm where you are now, but behave and act like the realm where God is taking you to next.

Do not allow your appearance to limit you from your destiny because your behaviour affects your becoming. So do not behave by conforming to the conditions of your current situation.

Hope is the secret of joy, so I will rejoice and enlarge my heart with joy.

A woman of hope is a stranger to the tension of anxiety.

What you refuse to welcome is not permitted to sit with you; I command you, spirit of depression, to disappear now in the mighty name of Jesus Christ. Now you say it and unseat depression from your body, mind, and soul because the Spirit of God has taken occupancy.

Once joy commences in the morning, praise takes over; I am joyous when I wake up in the morning because I don't take it for granted that it is the mercy of the Lord that brought me into the dawning of a new day.

Inspiration is the key you need to innovate.

Before you find what you like, do something you found out that you like doing until you find what you like.

The Holy Spirit would first find you busy with your business before He gets you busy in His business.

Insights without inspiration limit the greatness of your next level-up, so embrace opportunities if you want to change your levels.

Those who face challenges do not die of the challenges but defeat the challenges and challenge the challenges to death.

There is no big man in the pursuit of life; remain small in the eyes of God and allow God to make you big in the eyes of men.

To be a leader tomorrow, you must lead today, so decrease your size, and God will increase your height.

My father once said you go hiding only when you're not doing the right thing. Now I know the wrong things make us hide away.

I have an abundance of joy, and I am free to distribute it to whosoever God leads me to.

I am created with love and wired to be wonderfully weird in the world.

Until you understand the purpose of your creation, the vision will appear blurry, and the walk will seem wonky.

A person's voice can only be echoed by another and as the voice of the person who already has a voice. Rather, teach them how to voice things out than to be their voice as long as they are still alive to represent themselves, or else this act will not be respected more than the group or persons who stole their voice in the first place.

If you want to help people to find their voices, first teach them to speak out; then teach them to speak up. Everyone has a voice and has the right to demonstrate their freedom of speech. If you keep speaking on their behalf, you are part of those stealing their voice.

Everything done in its season is seasoned to taste better.

A book is your invitation card to get your invitation booked into a conference.

Everything is prepared ahead of TIME. God just happened to walk into it on TIME as God is ahead of TIME; hence His TIMING is always right.

God is what God is and not what we think He should be like. His benevolence should not be taken as a weakness because He is a righteous God who will judge both the living and the dead.

If you can't tell the difference between when you were in the world and when the word got into you, check if you have fully understood what it means to give your life to Christ.

Some people hate God because they do not understand that He already loves them and that all they need to do is to accept His love before they can experience His love for them.

The hospital is a rehabilitation centre where people go to recover, while the church is where people go to be healed.

I got my healing first before I was made whole.

You can steal my right to speak about my rights, but you can never steal my right to write about my right of speech.

Increase your trust in the word to validate your praise.

The more I know God, the more I understand myself; the better I understand myself, the more I see God in me.

They say there is no almighty living God, but they know that there is a creator – the almighty living God – and disprove those who say there is a creator (the almighty living God).

Firewood can never catch fire without a matchstick to be scratched to create the flame.

It is gainful to pray for one another because what you put in the basket is what you take out of it in multitudes.

The will of God is for us to share with one another. There is love in sharing, making love the greatest of them all.

'Soro Soke' is the generation born to talk.

When you hear them say you're too polite, you know they have been trying to fight you but don't know which angle to get at you.

Young ladies, don't open the door for afflictions; shut your legs.

Give love a meaning. Love is when you don't have it all yet are still deeply in love.

Faith is an invisible force that forces things to be visible.

Man disappoints, but God appoints because when God speaks, He has the capacity to contain it, unlike when man speaks, because he has the ability to facilitate it.

God does not need a man to complete what He has started. He is the Alpha and the Omega.

The crying heart of a mother in the garden is louder than the howling monkey in the forest.

When a pin falls on the eyes, it sits on top of the brain; that's why it's called a body. Hence, even a toothache can paralyse the nerves in the whole system of a man.

Be careful about who you befriend; sometimes the ones kissing you are the ones killing you.

Quietness is attractive. Silence is violence. Strangers can be dangerous, but a best friend in a day and a best friend from childhood can be enemies for life.

Only a prostitute can derive pleasure from having sex with a broken-hearted man.

The new peace is silence.

If I look like a flower, then I am.

Busy brain; lazy mind.

Only a brilliant parent feels like they have done overtime at work while minding the children at home.

The best thing about going away is coming back because there's no place like home as home is where the heart is.

When the race is over, at the end of the lane, the clappers say, 'You should have told me you found it hard, and I would have been there for you.' The reality is you can only tell tales of hardship only after you have won the fight and after the winner has been announced – not in the ring because you never know; when the countdown is over, in the midst of the adrenaline, a single blow can still snatch the belt.

You either drop dead trying or jump over deadly traps, having tried, for what does not kill you makes you stronger.

It is so painful to talk about it but more painful to think about it and not be able to talk about it.

Being ashamed to talk about mental health is like acknowledging there's a head attached to the neck but dismissing the brain inside the head.

I can't get over it, and I can't get under it, but I got on and so got through it with Christ my Saviour.

My anchor, my amour, my strength – that's my God.

Never be ashamed of something you have no control over.

When it is your time to shine, no amount of bad words can hold you down. Hence, when it is time to fly, don't crawl; be blown into the air.

Wisdom is greater than rubies any day; those who know their God shall rejoice, not those who bow to men.

Your greatness is not what you have; it is what you give because if you have it and give it not, then you are a nothing.

If you are not in someone's league, don't try to attract yourself to his or her team; just wave, walk on by, and leave them be.

If you notice that you are always miserable, check your company and check yourself out.

Live and allow others to leave. Never stay where nothing measures higher than your worth.

A woman owns a house, but there's one room that belongs to the man, the television room with a large-screen television. The room with pots is hers because that's where passion is cooked, which is the foundation that prepares the heart to contain the peace that it pours out.

Never tell another that your pain is greater than theirs because God does not give us loads according to the sizes of our heads; rather, He gives us shoulders that enable us to lift the loads on to Him.

Hi, ladies! Please don't lose your lives to sweet gossip; keep sealed lips for sweeter lives.

Pain is not common from one person to another. Every kind of pain is a different kind of pain according to a different type of person. Each person goes through a unique pain, so it is better to say nothing to a person if you can't say a word of blessing to add joy to their soul.

Dear parent, do not destroy the future of your youth by introducing things of the world to them through the television box at such a prime age.

A praying believer is not a fighting believer, a faith-filled believer is not a fearful believer, and a faithful believer is not a beggarly believer.

What favour brings to you is better than what labour brings to you.

Beloved, don't underestimate the power of praying for others and thanksgiving.

Say hello to a stranger; you never know what danger you will get them out of by the train track.

The best thing about being a child is the kid inside who is ever inquisitive outside.

Be that beautiful stranger who wears nothing but a smile.

Be the first to ask your spouse what you can do for them.

Whatever a man calls his wife, that is what she will be to him alone. If he calls her a bitch, she will be just that to him, even with a beautiful bow just to crown it off. If he calls her a queen, she will wear her crown and treat him like a king.

Know your niche; better still, know who you are. You can't be doing all the things that all the people are doing out there just because it is the season and know not their origin. I tell ya, it's the fastest way to lose yourself.

OK, you got your eyes on a different kind of fish, but you're dipping into the wrong sea. Know your audience; then find out where they are, or you'll be swimming all over the sea.

Being a copycat is not a tool to increase sales. 'If God no give that market, ei no go sell o, so no carry go.'

If another man's fall is your uplifting, it means that you're a very weak candidate. When you lend a fallen man a hand to stand up, you will still be standing tall.

When you walk with a dog, you must learn to drag a bone from other dogs. Choose your path wisely.

Go the extra mile higher; it's never crowded up there.

Everyone you met today is fighting an unseen battle, so be kind or be quiet; both choices are polite, so choose one or look away.

Anger, resentment, or jealousy doesn't change the hearts of others. It only changes the one who carries such a load on their mind.

When God says He's got your back, literally lean back because He is fixing everything behind your back. When a man says he's got your back, actually look back because he could be pulling out your backbone.

The man whom God uses positions himself where God will see him.

Knowledge is power; wisdom is powerful. Ask God daily for new wisdom each day as there are new challenges daily.

Distinguish yourself from others, even if they call you crazy. If you know where you're heading, keep calm, look forward, and carry on, going straight.

When you are looking at the beauty of a person, do you start looking from the outside, or do you look into their soul, which is the inner man and the real personality of the person?

I see a reason to live. I see light. I see life. I see. Lord, Lord, Lord, I see love. I see long. I see length.

When faith comes alive, fear dies, and when fear dies, life springs forth.

Propel yourself to elevate so you too can be saying, 'Thank you, Father, for making my vision bigger than depression.'

There's no abstract silence in a girl's mind. I only go where I'm wanted.

Thank you, God the Father, for giving me the spirit, not fear; I'm calm in the storm still.

After the rain comes the sunshine. Beauty is not measured by short sight, and nothing is hidden under the sun.

Happiness comes from your own human efforts, but joy comes from Christ the Messiah.

Marriage without trust is not like cancer, but it is cancerous because it is infused into the blood stream each time there is anxiousness because of the lack of trust.

Hear not the voices of strangers; rather, rest assured when you hear the 'I AM That I AM'.

Happiness is from the outside of a person and reliant on things attached to other substances. It is temporary because when the source of the supply is cut off, happiness is drained off.

Joy is within and of surplus; hence, it has the potential to be refilled from the same source of its internal supply. It can only be cut short if attempted to be stolen by an intruder.

Only deep thinkers can pull out the deepest thoughts of the mind. Stop to think; don't jump.

Launch on hope today. God is not a God of coincidence; if you kill yourself today because the enemy blindfolded your eyes so as not to see God's love, God can send your angel to turn your lights back on so you can live on.

When you get to the end of the track, don't jump! Choose life and be determined that life goes on.

Some may get annoyed by the truth being said. It is OK; say the truth anyway, even if your truth sounds like a lie because they have never been in the truth. Remain in the truth anyway.

When your best is not good enough for them, reverse your best to yourself.

If only you can see what sorrow does to the body inside, you will rewind your joy and rejoice.

Don't get carried away by the clappers; some clap to clap you off the stage. Remain focused.

Mind your step; an angel does not land twice from heaven for the same occasion. Once you miss it, it's gone forever.

Be the person who would be good enough for the person you expect to be as good as.

The heart of a man is wicked, just like the Father rightly said, but the Father also said that we should forgive them so that we can live.

Different strokes for different folks – don't kill yourself over the opinions of others. No one but God knows how your heart beats.

Don't force your way into the mentality of others who especially visualise the issues of life from a different outlook to yours.

Your qualification will come to nothing if your edification is zero.

First, listen attentively to whom you want to hear before you start listening to them. The first two things they say usually indicate to you if you should continue listening to them or not. You decide.

Your presentation of yourself is an indication of whether your reception would be received well or not.

God himself hardened the heart of the pharaoh so that His plans for the Israelites would prevail. Let's learn to thank God even for the ugliest parts of our past because they have led to our beautiful future.

Champions are not made sitting down. Get up and match on.

Take time to discern so you're not quick to burn out.

If you've never starved for food, you will not know what it feels like to be hungry.

Men would intimidate their wives to gain control of them if they step over their boundaries. Meanwhile, a woman would use manipulation to gain her weight round the house by laying on a guilt trip for the man to submit to her wants.

Greater is the end than the beginning.

Living a life without growing is dying slowly without knowing. If you wake up every day and think outside the box a 100 per cent to be doing everything right 110 per cent daily, this means you are not adding something new to yourself

daily. This indicates that you are not evaluating yourself for a change, which, in turn, would leave you living a life without change, equal to the lack of an increased and enhanced life.

You ask in prayers and then listen in waiting. He who has ears, let him hear.

If you are not satisfied in the presence of God alone, you're never going to be filled with the presence of God and so may miss it when He speaks.

I AM your arm for strength.

I AM your eye for protection.

I AM your ear for prayer.

I AM your future for destiny.

I AM your will for faith.

I AM your gift for provision.

I AM your heart for love.

Dare to write a word each minute. You will discover that you have written a line from a page in a chapter of the book you hide inside of you. Write a line per hour, and it would lead to you writing a page a day, which would bring you to completely writing the chapters of your book in a couple of months.

I am a work in progress in the process – still processing.

Chapter IV

 EPIC POEMS BY MERISHA

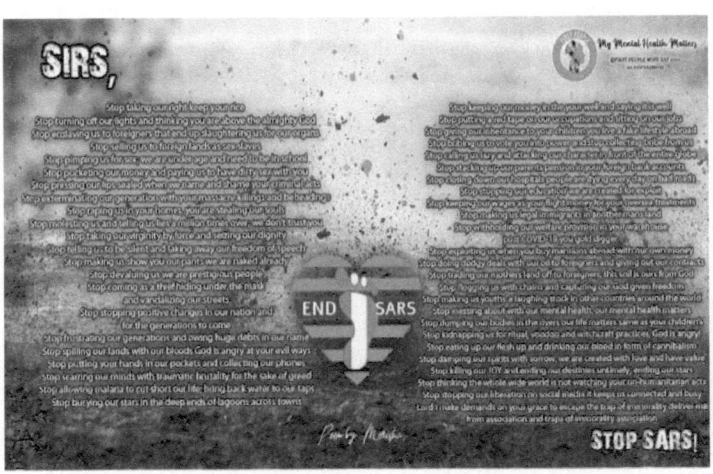 **Poems**

The protest End SARS, which began in Nigeria and went global, was a protest that brought me outside in the 2020 London lockdown. To be honest, I did not stop to ask God if I should go as I felt I was led to go, especially because on 13 and 15 October 2020, I received revelations from God about this movement in a very powerful dimension.

On 20 October 2020, at about 6:50 p.m., at the Lekki Beach toll gate in Lagos State, Nigeria, it was said that the Nigerian army opened fire on her youthful citizens who were peacefully protesting for their right to be heard by their government for a better Nigeria. I was taken aback on hearing this. **This date, 20/10/20, has been marked globally as the Lekki Massacre, the day that Nigeria murdered her own citizens on its own soil.**

I cried helplessly when I saw the news unfold. First, I cried, but I did not know why I cried, and then I cried for the Nigerians, and third, I cried for myself. I became angry because I could not do anything about what was going on or change any of it. Then I got upset because the most great, influential people in the world who could do something about it did not show any interest.

I picked up my pen and paper, and while still sitting by the window near the radiator, I began to write down my thoughts:

> *The system operating in Nigeria at the moment and for many years is cooperative slavery to entrap Nigerian citizens all over the world. This system is more favourable for foreign associates who are the major beneficiaries of the suffering of Nigerians.*
>
> *We are not here to entertain anybody! The entertainment box is the biggest screen in most houses.*
>
> *How come everyone who calls himself or herself a Nigerian is not bothered but would get on board for a better Nigeria? I could see the black British youths are very zealous with hope to go home to a place in Africa. I wonder – how come I have not seen any consoling statements from Boris Johnson with the large amounts of hard-working Nigerian citizens in the United Kingdom?*
>
> *There are other very influential voices in the world whom Nigerians will appreciate seeing join them in solidarity with their grief. I*

personally was hoping to hear from members of the British royal family, especially because of their voluntary duties in line with the work they do as humanitarians and their passion for Africa.

Nigerians all over the world joined the march for Black Lives Matter following the police killing of George Floyd in America on 25 May 2020. Now Nigerian lives matter a lot, especially because even on their own soil, they are not allowed to breathe. So where is the guarantee that they would be given their birth-ordained right to breathe and voice out their opinions in another man's land?

Mind you, all lives matter, but where is everybody?

The collective voice of very intellectual Nigerian people is needed now more than ever to demonstrate solidarity with the people of Nigeria because the Nigerian youths – heroes – are being gunned down to the ground for using their voices to dispute issues that have been holding down their destinies.

On 21 October 2020, ex-president of America Bill Clinton tweeted, 'I am deeply concerned over reports of violence in Lagos and urge the Nigerian government to engage in peaceful dialogue with the #EndSARS protestors for police reform and an end to corruption.'

Following this nudge from Bill Clinton to President Buhari to attend to the cry of his people in Nigeria, I saw President Buhari's brief appearance on TV, and based on Buhari's body language, he was emotionally disconnected. Watching this made me feel so disappointed to observe how careless the appointed person to lead the Nigerian people seemed, not bothered by the death of civilians.

Fast-forward to April 2021, I learned that President Buhari arrived on the soil of the United Kingdom, England (London), for his routine medical checkup as a normal checkup is a misfit.

Why are so many people still scared to talk when they are dying for not talking already?

RAINBOW GLOBE

Poem by: Meisha Merisha

Dear Lord,

My Father' who at in Heaven., But also here with me on Earth.

I see your Rainbow everywhere all around me.

Out of every person, I see the sings of you.

On every home, I see your signs.

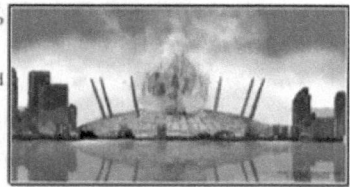

Even on the rooftops of rooted tress, I see your signs like floodlights weaving on the streets with the love of the father.

I see your signs on the grounds and I see it on the sky,

I see your beauty everyday in everything I touch.

Everything you created I see is beautiful, and I wear it everyday on my fabrics.

I see the rainbow signs beautifully sweeping across the nations of the earth and

drawing everyone together as one with the love of the father.

You show me your beauty in every person you created; big, small, large and thin.

I see you connecting all man, woman, boy, girl, young, old

Infant

Back to you through your Rainbow.

Your Act of Love to grant Peace to the World;

Is in the Ark so that no man would perish,

But that all men would return back to you in repentance at your presence.

Though you are patient in your ways...

In a way that I can see your ways are not my ways but I mirror to become as you are. So who I'm I to condemn those that you want to save through the body of Christ Jesus, my Lord and Personal Saviour.

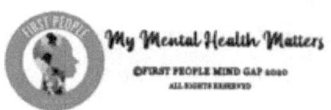

This revelation on 13 October 2020 came in two parts. The first part I saw was a fire burning in the clouds, as seen the image description of the 'Rainbow Globe' poem. 'What has fire got to do with the clouds in the description?' was not a question I found myself asking; rather, I was in a blaze – not that I was burning, but I was very gripped by the scene. The fire burned for a short while, but the intensity of it had a long-lasting effect that made it look like the burning went on for days.

The fire did not burn me, but I knew my emotions had been tampered with, and so this left me very espoused and hurt. My spirit had left my body, and it was wandering round an unknown ground. I was captured by death but released to come back to life. When I saw my spirit walk back into my body from the dead, I began to sing a song from the forest where I walked barefoot – but not before I saw the blood droplets from the sky, which was the second part of the revelation.

On 15 October, there was a great outburst in the sky. It was a bubble of blood drifting down from the sky. I saw it fade from red to pink, and then it formed into balls in different colours of the rainbow. I then saw a great chain of people on the ground – among them was me – in tiny little circles, gathered together, holding hands while lying down flat on the ground in a uniform circle.

The ground was wet; we were by a water fountain that gushed out water with very powerful force, like a shower engine with a weapon of destruction. Everyone lay low and stayed still – starting from tiny to big, bigger, and biggest – all intertwined in a bow, leaving the greatest or tallest among all undistinguished.

I walked while singing a brand-new song which the Lord had put in my mouth and which I sang non-stop. I woke up still singing the song, which you can see in the image of the 'Rainbow Droplets' poem. The Lord caused me to sing a new song, having shown me His face and mercy. Yes, I saw the Lord, for in my pain, He showed up, and in death, He rescued me.

I was surprised to learn of the End SARS protest, although I remained passive with any engagements. I was rather gobsmacked to discover the Lekki Beach killings of the youths, which happened on TV. I am still astonished that I was a part of that movement and that God chose to revive me even at a time when I didn't identify as an influencer of the protest or wasn't even associated in any form of significance.

Still, I am coming to understand how God would have chosen me to be a part of that experience and many more outpouring revelations from this encounter. I saw why it felt natural for me to join the protesters in a march to 10 Downing Street, Great Britain, because of the revelation. In it, I did weep bitterly, not because of any physical pain per se but because of deep emotional trauma.

I wept frightfully with a fearful embrace. Even if I had an awareness that God had saved my life, I was not fully conscious of the depth at which the angels of God had stood on my behalf to remain alive. It wasn't until I rose up that I realised God had given me another chance to live on earth, not for myself alone but for Him who had shown mercy on me as well as shown me that there is indeed eternal life.

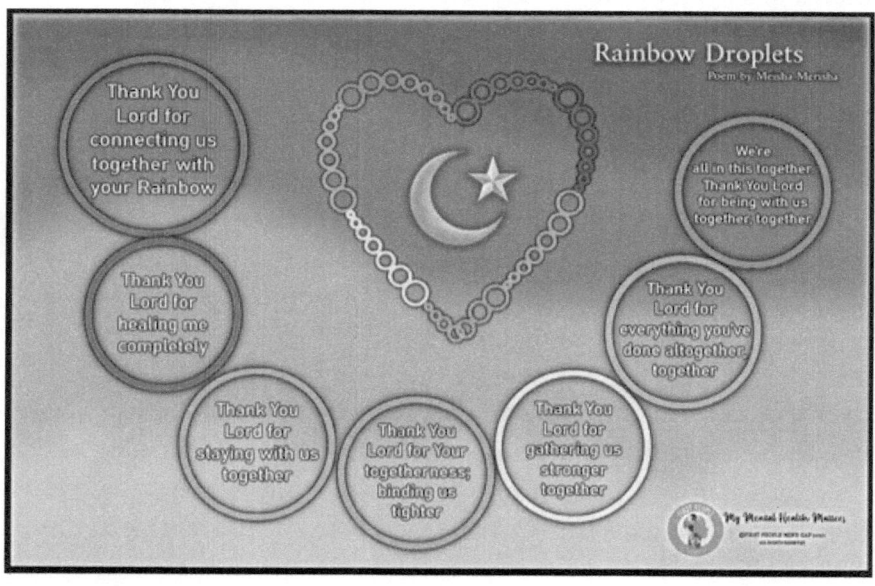

On the early morning of this day (15 October), after receiving the revelation, I stepped outdoors for my routine walk. Whilst I was outdoors, I saw a young moon and a bright star (Venus) next to the thin-shaped moon in the very early hours of the morning. I remember the repeated comments of my creative partner when I described the art piece of these poems, 'Rainbow Globe' and 'Rainbow Droplets': ***'Oh my god, are we all going to burn in hell?'***

An unrecognised laugh came out of me at hearing the words from a weary voice. I don't know why I laughed. I still cannot tell how I could reply with a laugh. Still, our responses are not always calculated, and not all laughs come from a place of joy. Still, holding on to the same conversation, I heard a loud cry inside of me with a shout saying, *'Go and tell them!'*

This time, what the Lord has continuously been saying to me since 2020, however, is that there would be His presence in the nations across the earth, full of His wisdom, through the rainbow. So do not condemn them who use it for evil, for they will be converted through it and drawn back to Him. It is the work of believers to use the rainbow to bring lost souls back to Him. While many are posed to be against Him, they need to be won back to Him but first need to feel love through the warmness of those who claim to love Him. Many who wage war against Him are depressed and ignorant and so searching for love but are falling into the devil's hands; the devil is using them for his evil work, not for good but to destroy them.

I returned home from my walk after giving praise to God in the open air. Indoors, I bowed my head, gave thanks to God in prayers, and prayed for the nations across the earth, as seen in the image of the poem titled *'Rainbow Globe'*.

These revelations were heard, noted, converted into poetry, and documented before 20 October 2020, the day of the Lekki shooting.

The significance of the Lekki shooting in both the 'Rainbow Droplets' and 'Rainbow Globe' poems is that the Lekki shooting was heard globally and across the nations of the earth. This ordeal led to the involvement of most of the nations of the earth in the End SARS protest. The relationship between the poem and the theme described here can be seen in the actual title of the poem – 'Rainbow Globe'.

◌ **Email Preview** ◉

15 Oct 2020,
09:50

This is a sketch of the rainbow heart droplets in the 'Sky' poem.

The drawing is of seven rainbows coming together in the sky in a heart shape. The rainbows maintain each line of their own colours but in

an outburst of droplets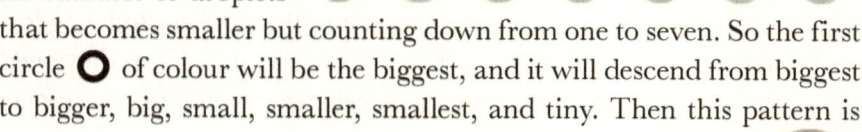

that becomes smaller but counting down from one to seven. So the first circle ⬤ of colour will be the biggest, and it will descend from biggest to bigger, big, small, smaller, smallest, and tiny. Then this pattern is

repeated seven times over for all seven colours of the rainbow into a heart shape that connects all as one.

In the middle of these heart-shaped droplets are rainbows, and after the first three rainbows, before the last four rainbows . . . right in between the gap will be a young moon and a very bright star right beside the moon, but the star will not be inside the moon or on top of the moon. It will be placed right beside it, as seen in the image I sent you of the top practice drawings of the rainbow droplets coming together.

This is the second poem you will work on, please, but let's finish and complete the first one first before going into this so that my head does not get inundated with the workload. I still have other creative works that I'm pressing on with, so I don't want to be overwhelmed with it all.

Tue, 13 Oct 2020,
07:07

The reason I'm writing this email is to let you know that I have written a new poem this morning.

The poem will be copied into a circle ⭕ in a circle ⭕ in a circle ⭕ in a circle ⭕ in a circle ⭕ in a circle ⭕ in a circle ⭕ SEVEN TIMES.

The drawing is of the Greenwich 02 Dome without the roof. The sky and fire replace the roof instead, and instead of the corns, it's

seven corns representing the seven colours of the rainbow

overlooking the rivers .

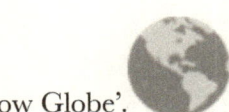

The title of the poem is 'Rainbow Globe'.

Please reply here via email, and I hope my email meets you well.

Kind and gentle regards,

Merisha Meisha

◯ Interview of DJ by CNN ◉

Below is an interview (paraphrased) with Obianuju Catherine Udeh, who is known by her professional name, DJ Switch, and who is an eyewitness of the Lekki Beach shooting that occurred in Lagos State, Nigeria. This interview was conducted by Becky Anderson from the CNN TV channel, who gave DJ Switch a chair to air part of her ordeal. However, from my perspective, I see how this interview reveals the correlation between the seven corns, as mentioned in the revelation, to the time the army arrived at the beach and to the number of bullets counted by DJ Switch that were seen on the scene of the shooting.

Becky: '*DJ Switch is now in hiding but is bravely joining us to speak about what happened that night. And we thank you for doing that. What has happened since? The videos that you posted have made you a target. There are claims that the Nigerian army has been trailing you and threating your life, even forcing you to flee the country. The army has denied this . . . saying that there are bigger fish to fry.*'

DJ: '*What I experienced that day was the worst experience of my life . . . Thanks for giving me your platform to continue to talk and share this story. The Nigerian army that is meant to protect us came with no warning. None. None. No representatives to come and speak to us first at least. They just came in, [guns] blazing.*

'*We heard gunshots from behind the toll gate because we were on one side of the toll gate, so we heard [gunshots] from behind them, with people running, so what we did was just to go back and sit down still and wave our flags. We believed that if we waved our flags, they would see that we are not here to cause any harm or any trouble but just to protest as it is our right to do so.*

'*There was no warning, nothing. People were just dropping, and I can't even explain that to you. It was such a chaotic scene that most times, I found it difficult to close my eyes without seeing those scenes replay on my mind.*

'*After they left, the Nigerian police came – SARS, to be precise . . . looking at the [uniforms of] the ones we could see and especially one man that wore . . . white. I don't know who he is, but he had like a small pistol . . . This man in white, he just kept shooting at us directly, and we were just running from left, right. That's the short of it, really.*'

Becky: '*[A] statement from the Lagos State governor highlighted that there would be change, stating, "Becky, I genuinely believe that there would be change for the following reasons. One, what had happened in Lagos is extremely unimaginable . . . Two, it was a [clear] call for all of us in government, especially in terms of understanding and realising the youths and what they truly want us to be doing. It hit all of us like a [ton] of [bricks] and assigned all of us a wake-up call."*'

DJ: *'With no due respect, I just [challenged] the governor of Lagos State to say the truth. They know the truth. Why not just come out and say the truth? Because it's been out there, their conflicting stories. Nigerians have died. This is not the time to play games. Families are looking for their loved ones. To be honest with you, with [regard] to me, I don't know how to feel because [on] one hand, I am grateful that I am alive today, but [on] the other hand, I don't know if I should say I am lucky because it is as if I am saying that the others are not lucky. It is time that we own up to the things that we [are] supposed to own up to. The government had a responsibility to the citizens of Lagos State, and he should say the truth.'*

Becky: *'[The] Nigerian president on Tuesday [vowed] to prevent a repeat of what had been a wider anti-police brutality protest through dialogue and through listening, he says, to all stakeholders. I just wonder – how does [his comment] make you feel?'*

DJ: *'To be honest, Becky, at this point, I do not hold what the president of the Federal Republic of Nigeria says to . . . heart. Nigeria is a dictatorship with a democratic face, and I think that is primarily to please the international communities. It is our right to protest on anything that we see damaging and demand for a change. The Nigerian government has used [force] from the beginning, when we were trying to infiltrate a peaceful protest with criminals, which did not work out, and then they moved to bringing in the ministry.*

'So the same government that says that they have [banned] SARS – and this is going on for five years now, where they keep [banning] the same SARS – is saying that he wants to have a dialogue? The same president has not even come out once to address the issue of the shooting at the toll gate. So no, Becky. I do not take his words to heart. We need action! We need change, and most importantly, we need accountability.'

Becky: *'You've said about this whole experience – and I quote here – "It is [a] cause for what I believe. Just . . . it is shock at the response of my government towards the people it is sworn to protect. It is courage to speak up no matter what and, for me, the will to see justice, accountability, and a change in Nigeria [no] matter how much is offered to me or [the] threats to me." Do you believe that change would happen in Nigeria, and how long do you think that you would need to stay in hiding for?'*

DJ: *'To be honest . . . the will is there. This generation – we like to call ourselves SORO SOKE. That means "Speak up!" Unlike the past, where they . . . oppressed* *our parents and misinformed our parents because we did not have social media back then. They owned the media houses and the newspapers then. But this is a different generation, and that goes to the end, where I believe strongly that Nigeria would change. It's not a sprint. It's a marathon. And now the Nigerian people, especially this generation, are speaking up!*

'The shock for me was to see that for the first time, something that gave me such [belief]. I never thought that I would see Nigerians come together with the same voice. Speak in one voice, demanding change and an end to police brutality. I never thought that our government – for the first time, they are seeing this – respond with inaction . . . seizing the passports of protesters, for example, arresting them, and chasing people out of their houses, out of town, and literally out of the country.

'I believe that . . . I have been given a second chance at this life. I don't know what would happen to me. I don't know what would happen to my carrier, all my bookings, and everything is gone. I don't know, but what I do know is that . . . I have this [choice]. I would use this opportunity to tell the story no matter the length, no matter the breath. I would use this opportunity to tell the story.

'My hope is to go back home. I don't want to be on the run anywhere. People think that I have . . . asylum. That is not the fact. But you can't chase down anything. Those things are not important. I want to be able to go home, but I want to be able to tell my story out of other witnesses under [oath], and then when I'm done, I can go home. If they want to pick me up after at that point, there's nothing to silence me . . . anymore. So if they still want to pick me up after that, they are welcome to do just that.'

Hungry London

Poem by Meisha Merisha

Have you thought of me since I walked pass your house
hungry
Do you recognize my face under your mask when you
peek into my eyes
Can you tell I observed you quickly crossing over the road
with two Tesco bags
Did you notice I opened my mouth to say you a hello' but
closed it up gain at once
Would you mind the gap if I stood on the edge of the
pavement
Could you tell I waited for you to walk on by as you do
and you did
Did you see me wear a smile when you wore your gloves
with a frown
Not a blink or a wave; still I'm famished, I saw you vanished in rampage for
food
Was I on your mind when you closed your doors and left me panting on your
doormat like a baby fox wondering where's everybody
Can you see me standing here naked; Posed vampish but dampish hair on
silky skin
How cold I felt, did you feel? As you hastily swiped my skin in grab for
tissues
Is it easy to spot the goosebumps on my body; not because I tremble from the
frost, but because you snatched the frozen seeded bread I held so close to my
chest with thoughts to feed the birds of the streets
Can you sense I seek to hide my face in the curve of my palm when I saw you
sanitize your hands after meeting my body with yours in your grab for bread
Still you keep the bread happily away form the birds
While I keep my smile till June allure of a sunny day in loop for the news
shopper
Will I not cry in wonder of such a solitary mews where there should be
solidarity in a time of uncertainty; I gaze up to heaven for my rainbow;
When you are locked in
eating, and I'm locked out twirling with the birds tweeting, I'll be the
rainbow in your cloud.

My Mental Health Matters

◐ 2020 ◉

Bishop David O. Oyedepo had prophesied that 2020 would be my year of breaking limits. Pastor Paul Eneche also prophesied that I would experience a drastic supernatural shift. I not only claimed this year as so but also worked towards it as an ambassador of God, walking into His supernatural ways.

Just before the beginning of 2020 and at my very entrance into this year, I began to get frequent messages from heaven. Some of these messages, if not most, were prayer-centred messages, and I believe that the more I was willing to accept the instructions, the more I received more instructions.

Once, I received the instruction to pray twenty-one prayers of thanksgiving, so I decided to dedicate these prayers to different countries across the globe. Almost immediately after I accepted and began this intercession, I heard God giving me a list of countries to pray for in this order: Nigeria, Canada, Britain, and so on. I told my eldest sibling to join me in this prayer as I maintained prayer as a lifestyle, but I began to receive stronger and more frequent revelations from God; the more I devoted time with God, the more I received from God.

The first message I received from God in December 2019 for the year 2020 was that in 2020, the earth would swallow a lot of people. After that, I began to get instructions from heaven to pray for people all over the world. So I changed my prayers from local to global.

I remember planning the Christmas holiday period with one of my church sisters who lives in Crayford, London. I would be cooking the big bird, and the rest would be on her. However, what was apparent to me from the conversation held on the day I went to her house was that during the prayer session, she asked me what my prayer request was, and I said, 'Pray for the world.' I would not forget the look on her face when she said in reply, 'What about the world? Should we be praying for youths, the church, or what?' – her face when my reply was 'Everyone'.

Coming into January 2020, in the first week of the year, I met up with my creative partner, who began to suggest to me that we should make a production on depression and death. However, by this time, I was going through various stages of anxiousness and experiencing anxiety attacks as a result of the message I had received in December about the earth swallowing a lot of people, but I did not know how. I could trace the reason why I was nervous as a result of this being revealed to me, but what I did not know was if I would lose any members of my family or friends among the people that the earth would swallow in 2020. As I was not sure if any of the people or I would be among those who would depart from the surface of the earth, this revelation was one that unsettled me.

It is true that I had to manage my own mental health first before I could support others with theirs. So I began doing some therapeutic artwork about my emotions. As I did, I paid attention to what sensations triggered my skin to react and my legs to move as if a live wire went through my veins. Surprisingly, more often than usual, these sensations occurred of their own accord without me being aware of the reasons underneath the surface of their reoccurrences.

Interestingly, my spirit was healthy, as was my mind, but my body was indicating that there was something I needed to pay deep attention to. I tried not to panic when the revelation replayed in my mind, but it was hard to control these electric vibrations/fluctuations. It is true that at the initial time of receiving this revelation, I did not know what to do with the knowledge. I had no idea how it would play out or at what dimension; it was incomprehensible.

I struggled to digest this information, especially for the reason that I had lost my brother in 2010. Now ten years onwards, another theme of death was apparent to me. This kept me adamantly active in search of ways to take better care of my mental health. Progressing, I read books on anxiety and phobias from both the spiritual and psychological bookshelves.

In January 2020, I disclosed to Ellien, my creative partner, that I would suspend the live production on death and depression until I had treated my own mental health. I also disclosed that the revelation I had received from God was about how the earth would swallow a lot of people in the year we had just arrived in, and although we had no idea what this message carried, we were equally both alarmed.

Each time I revealed to Ellien what God have revealed to me, she acknowledged me, and we both continued with our work. I worked with Ellien throughout 2020, and God has used me to show her that He speaks the affairs of His mind to me, which frightens me. He loves me and demonstrates how real He is, but I am only frightened in my love for Him.

In January 2020, the Holy Spirit began to paint the picture of the rainbow in my heart in numerous levels of depth. I was very intrigued by this; at the same time, I was curious as to what the metaphor was. Still, I went along with my fascination of the images, extending them beyond my mind. I wrote songs and sang them and emailed these back to myself. Just like a child, I awaited the Holy Ghost to show me what I needed to know next about the rainbow. Little did I know that this would soon become the symbol of the world connecting and painted all over the globe.

I saw the rainbow everywhere in my mind. What nobody else could see, God was showing me, and the Holy Spirit was taking me through it all the way, yet I had no idea where it was all leading. Still, these live visions grew beyond my mind to the point where I began singing about the rainbow. **The revelation of the significance of the rainbow symbol became obvious in March 2020 during the first British lockdown of the year, which was announced by Boris Johnson.**

◐ People's People ⊛

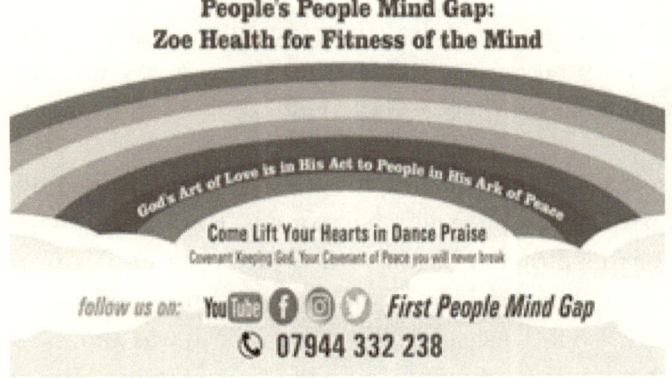

People's People Mind Gap:
Zoe Health for Fitness of the Mind

God's Art of Love is in His Act to People in His Ark of Peace

Come Lift Your Hearts in Dance Praise
Covenant Keeping God, Your Covenant of Peace you will never break

follow us on: You Tube ❶ ⊙ ◯ *First People Mind Gap*
☏ **07944 332 238**

On 28 January 2020, I received a message from God in a single word: **solidarity**. After I received this message from the Holy Spirit, I knew that God was still telling me something about people, even if I did not know what exactly. The word 'solidarity' said a lot about people, so I continued to pray for people of all kinds, but I wrote it down as I documented it, just for precision measures.

On Thursday, 13 February 2020, I was woken up in the very early hours, 2:00 a.m., by the phrase **people's people**. I tried to drift back into sleep, but *'people's people'* repeatedly sounded out from the Holy Spirit. Again, I didn't know what any of this meant, but it was a right 'Wake up! Wake up! Wake up!' I just had to wake up. All sleepy, I searched on Google, 'What does people's people mean?' However, the term 'people's person' came up, and I thought perhaps the Holy Spirit was telling me that I am a 'people's person'. I did not know what else to think of it, so I emailed it back to myself so that I could look into it when I was fully conscious.

Amazingly, the following Saturday, 15 February, I went to evangelise in the London borough of Bexley, right in the centre of Bexleyheath High Street, with a believing sister called Faith. At the end of this trip, I was making my way home when I saw, for the first time, the vibrant Metro Bank poster with the writing 'Award-Winning **People-People**'.

At best, shock gripped me at the sight of 'People-People' out of the blue. It was as if I was still sitting under the feet of God, receiving the second dimension of the first part of the revelation I had heard clearly at 2:00 a.m. on 13 February 2020. It then occurred to me that I had to take a picture of this poster just to validate the accuracy of God's lead, even if I did not quite know where I would land.

I could still see people moving around the streets, going about their errands, but I stopped hearing their sounds. Rather, as I snapped a few pictures of this poster, I began to hear a thousand-plus words in my mind, such as 'This kind God!' and 'It is you again' and even 'Should it be "People's People" instead of "First People"?' It was almost as if I knew already that it was God, but I wanted to be sure it was Him appearing to me again to confirm that He is with me always, even when I embrace or fail to embrace His presence.

Standing amazed, I stared at the poster until I came back to my senses.

Then I heard Sister Faith say, 'What is it? You're taking a picture of the poster?'

As I turned to depart from the scene, I heard someone call out my name. It was a student from the college I had once worked at as a student support worker for students with emotional needs. Lillian, one of the students from that college, recognised me; even though she was not among the students I had worked with, her surprise and excitement to see me thrilled me. She exclaimed how surprised she was to see me and said that she believed that it was God's doing as she was not meant to be in the Bexleyheath area. After I reassured Lillian that there's no coincidence with God, Lillian invited me to a women's conference, which was scheduled for the coming Saturday, 22 February 2021.

At the conference, I met a woman called Sharon. Sharon led the prayers on the outline, whose topics were around breaking stagnation to fulfil our life's purpose. I watched carefully when she spoke because her utterances made me listen, and her speech got my attention, so I stayed close to her until the end of the meeting.

Sharon offered to drop me off. On the way home, we talked, as we do, and from the conversation, Sharon found out that I had a business called First People and that I had recently received a revelation on 'People's People'; what happened next was beyond words and expression.

About that, I mentioned that I had a T-shirt line. Sharon also told me in excitement that she had an embroidery machine in her car boot which she had just picked up from outside London for her brother, who had a T-shirt-making company. This was not a coincidence; I know that with God, there is no coincidence as everything happens for a reason. Having said that, what was brilliantly unexpected but destined to occur was the discovery that the name of the company that had sold the machine to Sharon was called People-People. Funnily enough, as surprised as we both were, it was a delightful moment captured as we both laughed hysterically, looked at each other, stared back at the name of the company, and then said, 'Oh my God. What's going on?'

Right then, I concluded that there is more to this 'People-People' than I'm embarking on. Even if I still did not know what God was saying to me in full, the sequence and frequency of these 'People-People' messages and signals put me in a hurry to do what the Lord was prompting me to do. This was to gather people together and begin to give praise in His name – at least the first stage of it. I heard this accurately, and without any complacency, I began venturing into arrangements of how I could lift my voice in praise to God.

By 27 February 2020, I had printed out invitations in the same colours of the rainbow. I then began to look for a hall to hire for the event so that I could begin at least the first few sessions of its kind. On 2 March, I got a hall to begin my sessions, but just before I could announce the start date, the lockdown in England was announced. Before the world knew about the coronavirus, however, God was already showing me in different stages in His revelations the calamity; even if the revelations did not come at once, each stage came with a new order of instructions, which I tried my best to obey. Some of these instructions included reaching out to my family and neighbours, and even if they were not all easy tasks, I trusted the Holy Spirit to lead and guide me through them.

At the very start of 2020, the Most High God called me closer to Him, and I can never forget in January when God told me not to fight in this manner: **'Do not fight.'** When I heard this, I automatically translated this instruction as not engaging in any kind –physical, verbal, or non-verbal – with anyone, man or woman, boy or girl. This same year, 2020, was when I plucked up the courage and began to sing in my garden. This inspiration for me to sing outside of my cupboard and into the garden stemmed from my survival from a drastic case of domestic violence in September 2019.

God went ahead of time and began to take me through some rigorous healthy routines towards the end of 2019 on how to get 'COVID ready', but I did not know what it was until it became obvious, what God was doing in my life to prepare me for the pandemic ahead of time. God, so merciful, even took me through exercises and eating and drinking sessions ahead of the pandemic. He showed me what to eat, what to drink, and how to walk my way into a fitness walk ahead of the virus.

When the Holy Spirit showed me how to make my own citrus drink in early February 2020, I was reading something on my handset when the cookies on my phone caused something to pop up: 1 Timothy 5:23, when Paul tells Timothy not to drink only water but a little wine because of his stomach upsets and frequent illness. Citrus fruits are known to have many compounds that can help keep a healthy heart and other health benefits. I was dumbfounded but not discombobulated when I saw how God was talking because beside this was the image of a selected citrus which helped me know where the Holy Ghost was steering me to. I say this because for a moment, I thought, 'What is this scripture telling me? Am I to drink wine or what?' Then I saw a collection of citrus images which showed up very quickly, and I rested assured.

Soon after this revelation, I was excited because of the infinite presence of God's reality upon my life and the intensity of it. I could not wait to mix this drink, which tasted very delicious indeed; I remember taking a small portion of it into the therapy room and sharing with my therapist how it came about.

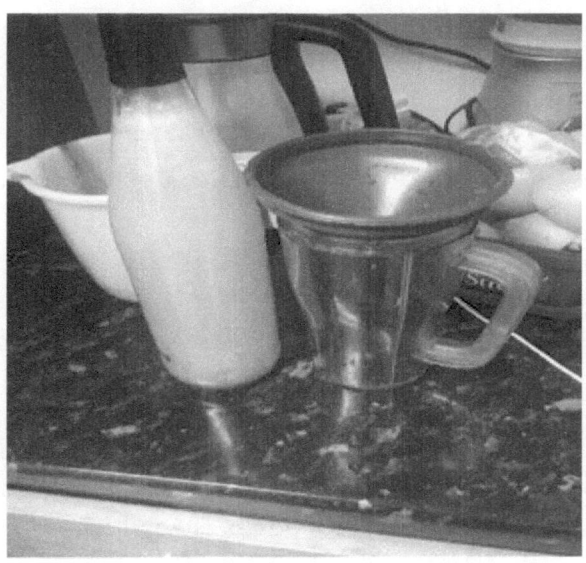

○ Churches ⊙

They fall in a very thin line of self-glorification in the name of praise.

There should be increasing testimonies of the salvation of souls won in the body of Christ and testified by youths and those who have been saved for the kingdom of God. My first true relationship with Jesus Christ, the king of the whole universe, began when my salvation was formed. The outcome of my salvation produced a wisdom I never saw in myself, and from then on, I began to hear more congratulations on my coordination, enlarging evidence of my relationship with Christ as an outcome of my salvation, to be multiplied from the orders of my testimonies.

Saying so though, a noticeable issue with the majority of existing leaders in the body of Christ is the attitude of most on the saying that *an old dog cannot be taught new tricks*. Therefore, they ignore the call to accept and replicate the testimonies and revelations of the new and upcoming ambassadors of God in the body of Christ, denying themselves from learning something new from what God is saying now.

Unfortunately, a million churches around the world are abandoning the gospel of Christ – the Messiah, the King, who is the only true living son of the Father – and are operating more as entertaining industries rather than structures of Christ for people to run into to receive their word from heaven for their salvation.

Meanwhile, for some of these churches, they deceive themselves, thinking that God is approving the way they praise Him. Remember Cain and Abel; when they offered sacrifices to God, Cain's sacrifices were not accepted by God, perhaps because he gave such offerings without a pure heart. Knowing that not all sacrifices, thanksgiving, and praise would be accepted by the Most High God, we should focus our teachings on the areas where the people of God are disobeying God and therefore making His presence not prominent in the midst of our gathering. I see this in the areas of sanctification of oneself, which is the temple, so that the life of the temple, which is the spirit of man, would be elevated by God almighty.

Something else I see these days is that most churches go on about building churches and making the buildings larger. They should aim to make the church of a person larger and pray for the saints across the nations of the earth to retain strength on the prayer altar, to keep praying for one another, not to faint these days while going on Christ's rescue mission of salvation for the unsaved souls among them, starting with members of their family. In the body of Christ is the blood of the son of the Most High God who died.

Why bother with the above statement of the children of God disobeying the Father?

The church is seen by non-believers as the biggest participant of disobedience to God's lead because of their lifestyles from the observation of their ordinances, both in physical appearance and inner utterances, not matching the word of God. Judging from their relationships with one another, in most scenarios, the absence of consistently demonstrating platonic love for one another leads to the conclusion that the lifestyles of most followers of Christ do not reflect the truth of God's abiding law, as evidenced in the life of one who drinks from the cup of He who is the true living water of the world. This leaves onlookers amazed, but amazingly, most of the people standing outside the church building looking from the outside are assumed not to be believers of the living God, believing in God more by the things they do in secret that are pleasing to God and derived from the things that have been cultured by their guidance.

The church/temple of a person is the component of the person that makes them sanctified and edified for God to use them in His kingdom. However, the sanctification of a person does not need to be approved first for the individual to begin their walk with God, for this is why God calls the unclean to be made clean and the unsaved to be saved and secured in His kingdom of light.

Yes, we the people of God are the church, and our bodies are temples. However, closing the doors of the church building has been very detrimental to all of mankind, especially non-believers of God, because in the midst of the COVID-19 chaos in 2020, a lot of scared people moved from one scary place to another scary place, with the doors of the church closed. Keeping the doors of the church closed has also brought about a lot of damage in the spiritual lives of believers.

Unfortunately, in 2020, the Boris Johnson government decided that the church is not a priority service to be left open in the COVID-19 pandemic. It failed to recognise that lives are saved in the church and that this is where sick people go to get healed; as the hospital provides beds and treatments, the church provides healing by the power of the Holy Ghost at work and in the name of Yeshua Immanuel.

As an effect of this action, your natural mind would never understand what the Spirit of God is saying until you dig deep. If you want to know yourself better, dig deeper into the things of God and allow your soul to receive Him; you'll find real peace that no man can give you and that surpasses all human understanding.

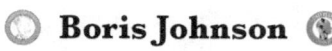 Boris Johnson

The 'Thank you, NHS' weekly claps by Boris Johnson were happening on my street, but at the time, I was giving glory to God. I believe that my life is sustained by the almighty God, not the NHS. This is what I believe, and without any compromise, I will not serve another god imposed on me in any other name.

However, I kept on getting revelations about Boris Johnson from God, and the instructions from the Holy Spirit were that I write him a letter. For me, this was not one of the easiest instructions to obey because I was writing to the prime minister, but the longer I left the letter unposted, the more I fell into disobedience. So the sooner I posted it, the quicker I fell into a greater peace.

Letter to Boris Johnson

Dear Prime Minister,

I am writing in relation to the current coronavirus situation, which has continued to be a threat to the human race globally.

From my observations of and conversations with people, it is true that a lot of people are apprehensive of the transparency of this new and invisible disease called COVID-19 as well as if it is an airborne disease or not because of the confusion of how we have to wash everything that comes from the shop.

I am very privileged to be able to write you this letter because you are my prime minister and you are a people's person, yet you are the most powerful man in Great Britain. As Britain is one of the most powerful countries in the world, this means that you are also among one of the most powerful men in the world, and as you are my prime minister, I have looked up to you to call the British people together for solidarity, and you have been doing so.

I am very delighted to see you have recovered from the recent attack of COVID-19 and to see you have resumed your presidential duties. I am also particularly proud of the way you have shown your appreciation to the NHS staff who have been trying their best to maintain the lives of their patients. However, sadly, the NHS staff have also been dying from this disease, so my question is who is protecting the lives of the NHS if the NHS are saving the lives of the people who are saving their own lives?

It saddens me to hear the announcement of the number of people who have died around the world caused by this invisible enemy. Most have referred to this as a demon that has no respect for anyone because even famous and wealthy people have been reported to be killed by this single disease.

Sir, I am aware of the national claps for the NHS which you initiated, and people have been following this ritual. Even up until now, the claps are still going on, and while this is to congratulate the NHS for their act of bravery, I noticed that the rainbow has also been connected to this activity. Again, this is very encouraging, and I can see that the people are doing what you've instructed to keep themselves safe and support one another while practicing these measures. Still, I cannot help but notice that this has brought up a lot of questions and confusion for children in Christian families about the significance of the rainbow and what the rainbow really mean to the nation.

These children of the Christian faith are confused as to what the rainbow means to the world, especially now, and they are asking a lot of questions about the rainbow of God and the resurrection of Jesus Christ, who brought solidarity to the world because His blood connected every man to God and declared that we are all one in Christ. God gave us Jesus Christ as our healer so that we do not have to suffer untimely death, but first, we have to believe, and there are a lot of believers in the world, most especially those who are working in the NHS.

The origin of the whole human race is from the provenance of God, so God has the power to preserve the lives of the people He created by Himself. So from biblical days, God provided the church for the people as a place of refuge to uphold the world by the power of His word; this is what heals the people from both physical and mental illnesses and cancer diagnoses when they call upon God with faith. Over the decades, most British people have been beneficiaries of the healing power of God, with frightful testimonies of supernatural healings. In most cases, what doctors have pronounced as having no hope, giving up on the individual and leaving them to die, prayers have brought back to life. I can say I am one of the people to testify this because in 2001, when my life support machine was turned off and I was left lifeless, it was prayers in the hospital that brought me back to life today so that I can share this testimony with you.

For decades now, majority of the British people believe in God, and many others do not because they say God is invisible; others mistake it as a religion rather than a relationship because of the lack of understanding about how the presence of God preserves life. This brings me to inform you that in this season of isolation and lockdown, people are killing themselves indoors, and these stories are not being highlighted in the media; maybe after the pandemic is over, reports of these cases will come out.

My plea to you is that you organise a day where everyone can stand in front of their door and acknowledge that the rainbow is God's art of love in His act to people, which is in His Ark of Joy for the people, and this contains healing. These are a few of the mysteries of God that trigger miracles and testimonies from people all over the world with proof that God, although invisible, gives life. He has the power to preserve people's lives by healing them from all forms of disease.

The coronavirus is invisible yet killing thousands of people globally, and this pandemic has instilled a lot of fear, loss, and mistrust in the lives of many people all over the world. As a result of this, some leaders of the world are also looking unto God to heal their land. Donald Trump declared a National Day of Prayer on 15 March 2020, and other leaders around the world have pursued this approach. I believe that for an illness you can neither see nor beat with medicine, why not try God's intervention? For those who believe and for many NHS workers, there are many Bible-believing faith workers who are waiting for the day when they will be permitted to join their faith with that of their patients and pray with them for recovery without feeling like they have committed an offence because natural remedies cannot be used to fight against spiritual attacks. The supernatural only will defeat this type of attack.

For people, being in the health profession is already an activity for God because the will of God is for all men to have good health so that they can acquire wealth and prevent poverty and thus prosper in both kinds of health. There are a lot of believers who are constantly and secretly praying to God in their hearts for the healing of their patients, just like the nation prayed for your own recent recovery with bold and public declarations that you get well.

People of faith both in the NHS and all over the nation are now praying for the invisible healer to kill the invisible killer, but there needs to be an agreement with the leader of the people to enforce this power. This is just like in the days when the Bible was written about ordinary men in society who went to their governments to have them join God to heal their land, and God answered their prayers. These biblical facts have been well documented for the benefit of generations to come so as to build up their faith and also be cited as points of reference to use in the days of calamity – as is true nowadays.

The American geneticist Francis Collins, who discovered the genes associated with a number of diseases and led the Human Genome Project, said, 'Jesus is the greatest physician.' He also said that God gave us an opportunity through science to understand the natural world, but there will never be scientific proof of God's existence. So the natural mind cannot understand the realm of the supernatural, but there are many believers working in the NHS who desperately want to be given the freedom to exercise their faith without causing any offence. They want to see people recover supernaturally and the NHS to be saved supernaturally because there are some things that human power does not contain, and it will not be able to maintain certain challenges. For example, God gave breath to men so He can secure their breath; that's why supernatural healing is existing in abundance today.

It is my hope that with enough concerns towards the COVID-19 pandemic and the uncertainty that rises with the large number of people who are still very sick from it, with no vaccine discovered yet, your office will consider my pledge to announce a national 'Flag Your Rainbow' day in acknowledgement of the significance of the rainbow, which is God's promise to the world of His love and not to flood it again so that peace can be restored in our community and in the nations of the world.

I thank you honourably for taking time out to read my concerns. I am an active mental health activist in my community. I have also recovered from a long-term physical affliction – an invisible enemy of its own kind and of sickness and infection – which has taken me to the hospital several times over an eighteen-year period for major operations and complications wherein I myself have also been in a coma and under the life support machine, fighting for my life.

I am self-employed and work part time on a zero-hour contract supporting special needs schoolchildren to help them get to school from their homes and get them back to their homes from school. I am also developing a clothing business and platform on mental health matters.

I live in the London borough of Greenwich, and my full name and address are:

[address written]

I trust that your government will reply my letter and address my concern.

Most respectfully,

Merisha Meisha

Fight the Fight of Faith

Poem by Meisha Merisha

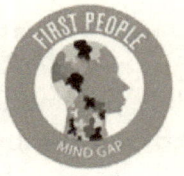

CORONAVIRUS, YOU ARE NOT FUNNY

Look How You Swiped Brexit In A Sec

You Became A Common Enemy To The Globe In A Month

And Your Best Features Are Anxiety

Drop Dead In The Name Of Jesus

The King Of Peace Is Living In My Lungs

A Fight Is A Fight And No one Wants To Die

So Be Gone, You Are Too Weak To Get Into My Street Still

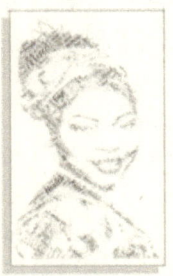

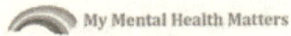 My Mental Health Matters

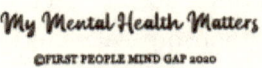

I don't know what is coming up for you as you read the poem titled 'Fight the Fight of Faith'. This poem is thought provoking and meant to trigger questions such as 'What can one do in times when stubborn challenges arise? Do you fall into fright or fight?' If you fall into fright, you've accepted defeat and willingly submitted yourself as a slave to fear in that battle; fear has overwhelmed you to think you're better off being eaten up by the challenge than dying trying to win. This is where your fright senses act as a response to the situation.

Meanwhile, your mentality if you choose to fight will be of faith because it is based on the truth that you believe in. You know that you will not die fighting because you are stimulated by the truth about the event you're venturing into, and empowered by the truth, you know about the source of your empowerment, which is the unfailing power of God that is backing you up.

Have you ever heard of a soldier who goes on a war front to fight for his country, and on his return to his country, he is being announced as the 'soldier defeated by his own people in his own country'? It is unheard of and would not be a clever thing to do because cowards never position themselves on the front lines, where they will selected as fit for war. However, it is more likely to hear a man of war being celebrated on their return, and even if a person dies fighting for their country, they are rather dignified with the title of 'hero' because of their act of bravery. It took them courage to step out and fight for justice in their country, but it takes a lot of faith to make this move so they will not be condemned.

This is exactly how God expects us to trust and believe in His integrity to deliver us, always knowing that He is too faithful to fail and will always show up to defend us and ensure that we are undefeated. However, the most important victory is salvation; this is when you are truly saved. By this, I mean when one rests assured that our souls are secured in God's hands and that we have a heartfelt relationship with God on a daily basis. Be mindful though that I'm not talking about going to a church building to serve alone; in addition, the most important aspect is serving God with our time in the church of our bodily temples. This is the 'living like Christ' lifestyle that I am talking about.

It is quite detrimental for a person to convince himself or herself that they are saved when they're not yet saved because of a pretentious attitude when it comes to salvation. This is what will allow the entrance of the Most High God into one's heart and begin a relationship to guarantee victory over any battle. How?

Imagine that when a soul is won on earth, heaven celebrates. Now imagine what will happen when that soul returns to heaven, what heaven will do; a party will be thrown, I've heard several men of God say. That soul would be crowned a conqueror when he/she returns to heaven, having encountered and engaged in the battles of life with the confidence that God is the mighty man of war who has gone ahead.

My conclusion on this note is that any person who is afraid of life after death is not sure of their soul reconnecting with God in heaven, and so that, for me, is an indication of their salvation being not quite secure on earth. However, this does not indicate that we live lives without divine wisdom − far from it. It is wise to not leave life to chance, to ask God for the wisdom that is needed for each and every day, and to renew our hearts daily before communicating with God day in, day out, keeping heaven guaranteed.

GONE VIA A TRACK

Poem by: Meisha Merisha

*Your sons and daughters, brothers and sisters,
mums and dads aunties and uncles, friends and
colleagues that you left behind; I'm in hope will
remember some of the memories you shared with
them.*

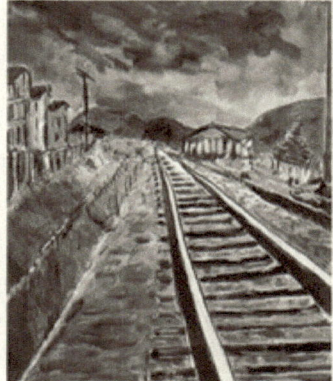

It had been an emotional ride drawing the words
out of my soul but the loudest quietness in my
silence would had been the real death of me, had
I not given me the space to express the anguish
that I felt in my mix feelings of a happy-sad
formed from the guilt to be conform as a survival
in the land of the living.

I did bury you in my heart for as long as I could
bear. But I could not stop my mind from bleeding over your soul.
Precious soul lost to a death crushed by pain so deep in the heart you felt it deep
pressed you to sleep' a sleep you wake no more.

How I longed to see your face breeze into the dawn from dusk till the sun sets on my
face, for the beauty of waiting in black' never fades off when the dullness of the dark
beams into twinkles of light to quench the dimness at the end of the day.

*The day is bright and fair but unfair is the day without you in it to grab a walk through
pass-holders lounge into my grad in grand style. I'm flabbergasted how life can brisk
so quick leaving one gasping for breath.*

*But now that I have buried you in the hands of the Lord, I can breathe again. A breath
of life I long to breathe and glad to say I smile as long as I live to breath.*

*I live and let the living live in peace with a dimples smile for you to know it doesn't
hurt so much the way it did when it did to see you no longer.*

Is painful to experience episodes of disappearing souls slip pass noiselessly to the
other side but more is the pain to be framed in this phrase and not able to give an
expression of it in words. These were the words that jumped out from my mouth as
soon as the tape pilled off my lips.

Rest in peace is the saying of many nowadays, but your eyes never witnessed the demon in the world today that came upon our lands and took many of souls who now sleeps till eternity in our community.

Many a' decade be my days far from yours.
Even so, I know I'll continue to pray a prayer that thy good Lord may have mercy on your soul as it continues to rest on in peace.

Piercing my face through the window before running around the garden in this quarantine, I see through the pigeonhole on the roof of treetops that 'My Mental Health Matters'.

I hear the sounds vibrating like a trump in a heartbeat sliding through the rivers, swimming across the Atlanta that made 'I' thrive against the rocks with my arms dangling on thin air.

The writing's fading away from my mind, my eyes sharp open gaping wide but I'm left on the floor discombobulated by the passers-by whose foot prints only I could see printing polka dots with missing body parts; struck suddenly on the neck by a knee weapon. I attempt to say from a gapped mouth...

I CAN'T BREATHE!

Desperately debating with self, trapped in an unfamiliar grounds, but I must breathe! Freely as its been given from above without CONVID or Men to seize my air as I run my race on a lone lane.

Gone via a track it seems like yesterday! Weren't you going for training on a train journey Johnny? I heard you cry safe journey but your journey was never saved sooner than it was my turn to cry save Johnny with an outburst.
No one heard my cries or saw my heart covered in plasters. So I dressed up my face and marched in front with feet moving backwards I don't know how I leaped forward if it wasn't for the ride on an angel's wings.

The train did run away with you, or did you run away with the train' a journey without a touch of light; I sat on a stool with a lit lamp to my feet tip- toeing and singing in the garden, beating drums that sounded like thunderstorm from the forest in alidimma; a good land but the few goods are due to land.

MERISHA MEISHA

I was covered in clay just before the rain came and washed it all away. I watched the people go in and out of their houses just to look at me dancing in the rain and I heard all that stoned the mad word to wound me. But they poured out their flesh through the crack on their broken windows because they had not known what it felt like to lose a piece of their heart on a sleeve you pull up but keeps rolling down.

I hear a knock on the door, approaching closer I see the car parked away from the block.
I thought I would lose my mind but I didn't.
I thought me absurd I'd lost the mind I held in my hands and carried with me to all the places I'd travelled to round the world but somehow I didn't.
I thought someone would care to care if any cared to see, but no one saw me because they all missed to smell the fear of life and death on the road that lead to the right was one, and to the left was another.

I stood amazed in the middle of the platform minding my steeps as I leaped on board bored steering at the blackboard on board with a blank mind.
I recognise the mask we wear everyday keeps changing but it never takes away the pain until we hand over the battle to the creator of life who can fill the void with love and close the gap that formed a hole hidden in the heart of a man that no one else could see. But he alone can feel every other beat that makes him want to jump out of the carriage, yet he keeps calm and ride on because he remembers the kids are waiting to receive the teddy and to say: 'I love you'.

I fought the thought for you and I for I knew to lose my life would be a lost of life indeed, of a life I did not create so I did give back to the creator who allowed me to cry in his arms, and He preserved my life that I forgone of a pain I could no longer bear from your disappearance and of me disappearing into a self I no longer recognised.

Gone too soon without your goods or a wave and a glance into your eyes nor blessed with your smile. I did question my brain' is it right to smile when I'm still grieving, or should I keep smiling with closed lips even if death hated that I did learn to smile again.

As death did not swallow up, I stay alive to tell my story today with a drop of tear and a smile; I smile, and I'm still smiling because you never stopped smiling and smiling is my present from God to show His presence in my life.

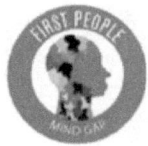

178

In 2010, I lost my brother to suicide. 'Gone Via a Track' is the path I used to empty out most of the stocked emotions that I had been trapped with. The poem is three pages long and like a mini booklet on its own, so I will say less in this session, but allow your mind to travel through a passageway I myself might have passed through in the days when I was numb to speak about it at all.

An open letter to my Pal

Dear friend,

As you open your heart to read my letter, don't be afraid to hold someone's heart, make them feel **good**; tell them that you **love** their smile.

Show **kindness** while raising mental health awareness on the act of Suicide. Be **patience** if they don't understand at first then apply **gentleness** when you teach them the reasons behind the missing souls that were stolen suddenly by suicide. But be mindful; apply **self - discipline** endeavoring to be none judgmental of their behavior on how they may react to this subject. Always be **faithful** when accepting other people's weaknesses and don't forget to renew your mind daily with the word of God so that your spirit man can be filled with **joy**. **This will give you peace of mind** and protect your serenity within your soul and will ensure your mental wellbeing is enhanced, so that you can have a fruitful day daily.

My Mental Health Matters
From First People Mind Gap
By Meisha Merisha

◯ **Prevent suicide. Be kind to one another . . .** ◉

*'People often ask me why I delete certain posts. The amount of
bullying and hatred I've had to put up with for three years . . .
I'm tired of looking at it. Be **kind**. Be gracious. We are
grown-ups . . . Stop acting like teenagers. Real women don't put
down other women.'*

—**Jessica Mulroney**, by Emily Kirkpatrick,
9 September 2020

The most beautiful thing about blessing a stranger with your **kindness** is that though you may never see them again, you have left them with a part of yourself. That is beautiful, and it would last in them for the rest of their life. It is true that they may not remember everything you discussed, but most likely, they will never forget how your smile made them feel at the time of your meeting.

In 2012, I collapsed on the floor of a British train after falling off an unbalanced side chair. What was apparent to me was that whilst I was lying on the floor in pain, I could see I was circled by the majority of people whose priority was to video-record me in my half-awake position on the ground. The only people I could recognise were the few people I was with from the beginning of my journey; apart from them, I did not recall the actions of anyone else asking after my welfare.

However, I found my legs covered up with one *'EVERLAST NY NEW YORK'* jacket I could barely recognise. When I asked whose jacket it was, I was told that a man put it over me to keep my decency kept in but was told that he left the train. What struck me at the time were his thoughts and act of kindness.

God's greatest commandment is love. Love, kindness, and peace are a major recipe for living a satisfying life. These elements of love, kindness, and peace, desired by men, interlock with one another because you cannot be kind to someone you are not at peace with, and it is impossible to heartily love someone without being kind to them. Consistent and generous love of life can be seen through a Christian in Titus (**a book in the Bible**). Paul the apostle writes a poem in summary: 'God's kindness and love are what [save] us despite ourselves'. Paul further illustrates that the churches should demonstrate that they are churches to become agents of transforming people's lives in their communities through peaceful living and showing devotion towards the work of Jesus Christ to all humanity.

ECHOs

Poem by: Meisha Merisha

They are antisocial towards you because of your peculiarity.

They never learnt to love, so all they preach is hate when you teach love.

They laugh at you because you have no child but they bear children they never care to raise.

They feed the street cat worms and watch the flies buzz round the dogs tail.

They put empty tins in the bin just to look at the sad on your face but find you merry.

They fight inside but laugh outside when they see you standing out.

They war with their flesh when they see you wear a smile on your face.

They wrestle with themselves when they see you chilling under the olive tree.

They want to see you tumble downwards when they see you climbing upwards but they fall flat on their face
as they see you rise to the top.

They pour insults on each other but mock you as soon as they see you walking by.

They act like they are having fun when they laugh at you minding your business but this makes them feel
better, away from their dysfunctions.

They lash out at the mysteries at work in you when they should learn to deal with their own miseries.

They swear to see you fizzle out but your star keeps shining brighter so they eat themselves up and drawn in
their own sorrow

They give you bad energy to make you their victim but your positivity keeps you victorious.

They look down on you but their looks can never pull you down because you are born blessed and bold.

They try to intimidate you with materialistic things but your giftings can never be measured to things that
are perishable.

They throw their rags over your fence to make you react but they hear your fame announced when the red
carpet is flung at your feet for you to step on stage.

They mocked you but your maker made you and in the end what they did mock of you became of them.

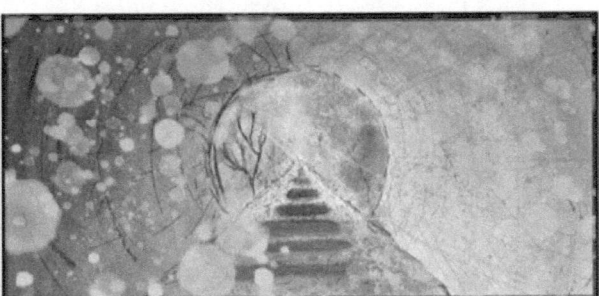

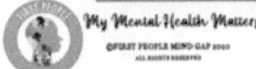

For over ten years, I suffered from antisocial behaviour from my neighbours, but the Lord has given me victory. If you've ever suffered such environmental hostility from people you live around who clearly have a problem with you being yourself and then begin to call you names to make you lose confidence in yourself, hang in there. The Lord is surely on the throne, and He will give you victory because the same people who called me mad yesterday have come to seek my counsel today.

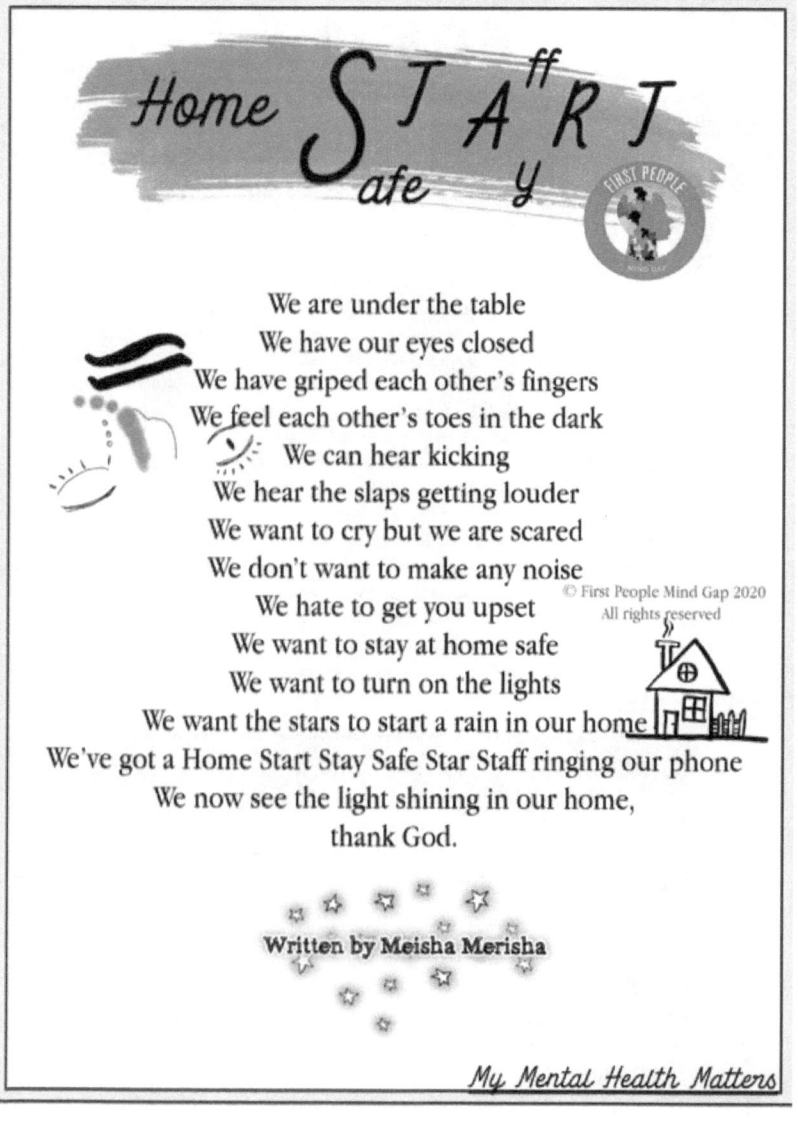

Home STAff RT Safe y

We are under the table
We have our eyes closed
We have griped each other's fingers
We feel each other's toes in the dark
We can hear kicking
We hear the slaps getting louder
We want to cry but we are scared
We don't want to make any noise
We hate to get you upset
We want to stay at home safe
We want to turn on the lights
We want the stars to start a rain in our home
We've got a Home Start Stay Safe Star Staff ringing our phone
We now see the light shining in our home,
thank God.

Written by Meisha Merisha

My Mental Health Matters

Domestic violence is classified as domestic because it's a type of abuse that occurs within a close network of people, at home, or within a family setting. There is nothing good about any type of abuse, but the worst side effect of abuse is either self-inflicted or forced upon as a result of the insults obtained from the abuse: death.

Once upon a time, I was involved in a relationship that unfortunately meant that I passed through certain types of abuse. Among all was physical violence, which led to the other person trying to kill me in a severe beating. I remember begging, 'Please stop. I could be pregnant. For the love of God, please stop. I may die.' There were other things I said, like 'I am sorry' and so on, but I remember a few bitter words they spat at me, and they were as good as telling them to a dead person, who, even at that point, would deserve better treatment.

It was a horrible ordeal. I could not believe that I could have been intimate with such a person, whom I thought a beast for a moment. In a gross but diluted description, I could see him sitting on top of me and yelling some horrific words, spat out of his mouth while he tried to tie me up with his belt until he found a rope. He swore the following: 'I will kill you, and no one would care about your dead body. This is Nigeria. I will kill you and whatever is inside you and throw your body in the gutter.'

It was then that I realised that I had signed up to live with a monster for the rest of my life. I wanted out but did not know if I would survive the beating or live to tell part of the story here today. I think the rest of the hostile words just passed through my head along with the blows, and all I could pant in my tender heart was 'Oh, God, save my life. Please save me. Please'.

Even if I did not deserve to live, those were my thoughts then. I wanted to remain alive to say, 'Thank you, God, for thinking me special and sparing my life should I see daylight after this dying state I'm honestly in.' I don't know how the miracle of when I stopped getting punched happened, but I can recall going through shock like I had never experienced in my life.

Surprisingly, I was hearing the song 'At the Centre of It All' by Eben play all over my insides after the attack, but I could not speak. I was searching for my voice, but I could not find it. I could see my ears were open, but I could not hear, and miraculously, my eyes were open, but I could only see what was right in my face, so my vision was blurry because of shock. God used this song to pump breath back into my system so that I could live, even if death stared at me.

At the centre of it all
It's you that I see
It's you that I see
At the centre of if all
It's you that I see

There is power in your name
Miracles happen in your name
As we lift our voice in praise
It's you that I see
It's you that I see
It's you that I see

Jesus, nobody else is like you
At the centre of it all, only you
I see, it is you that I see

You are bigger, bigger than the biggest
You are stronger, stronger than the strongest
You are higher, higher than the highest
You are greater, greater than the greatest

JESUS

Oh my god – this song gave me a free flight to heaven and back to earth so that I could appreciate a marvellous God.

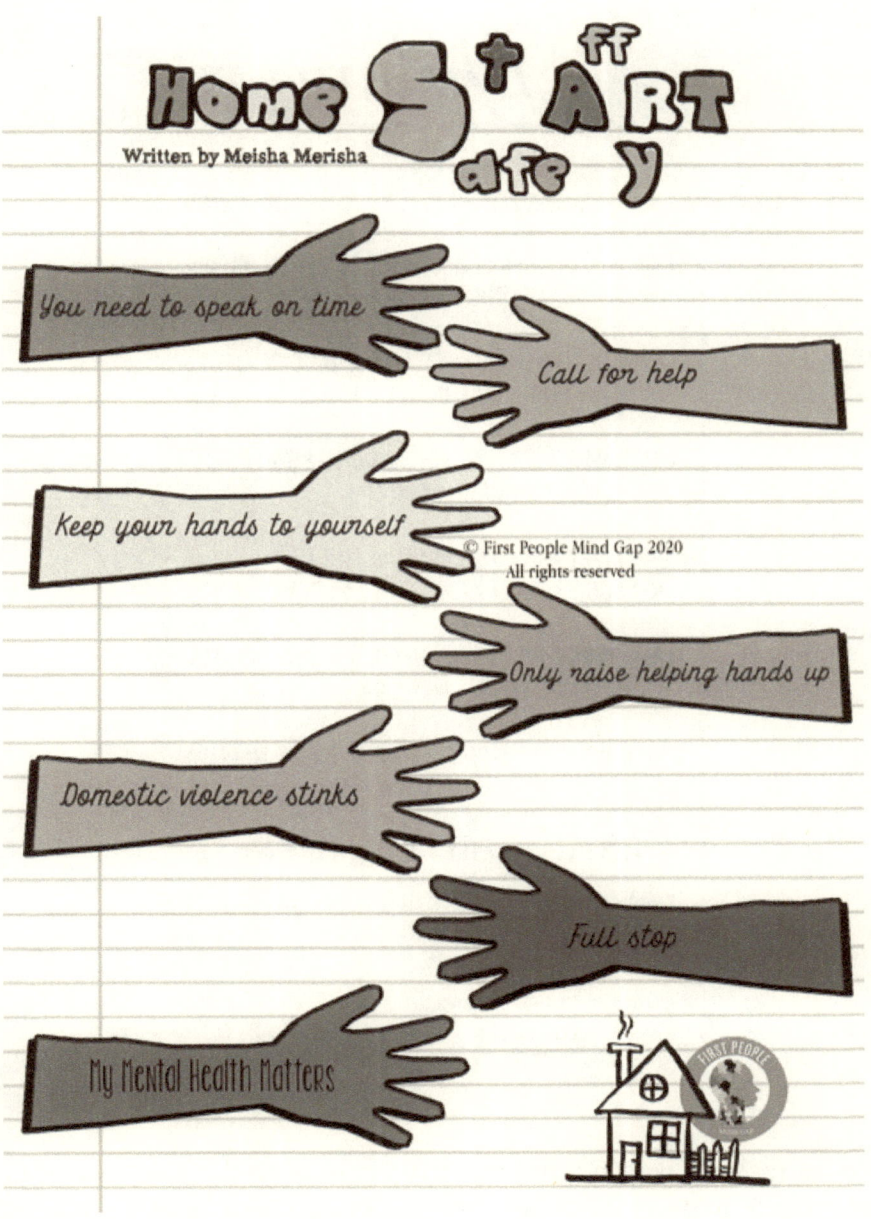

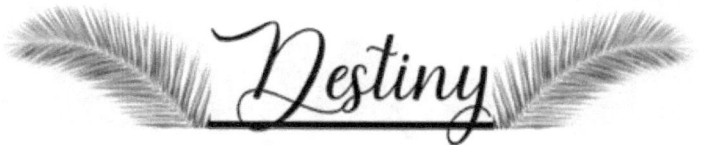

Poem by
Meisha Merisha

GOD'S ART OF LOVE IS IN HIS ACT TO PEOPLE ON HIS ARK OF PEACE.

NEVER PLAN WITHOUT GOD FIRST, IN YOUR FIRST PLAN FIRST PLAN WITH GOD.

FIRST MAKE HIS PLANS FOR YOUR LIFE THE FIRST PLAN OF YOUR LIFE.

IF YOU DON'T WANT TO FAIL, PLAN FIRST WITH GOD; IF YOU DON'T WANT TO FALL, FIRST PLAN WITH GOD.

LEAVE YOUR FIRST PLANS IN GOD'S PALMS PLANTED FIRST IN HIS HANDS.

IF YOU WANT THE WORKS OF YOUR HANDS TO PLUM UP LIKE THE PALM TREE.

FIRST PIN IT IN THE FINGER TIPS OF GOD

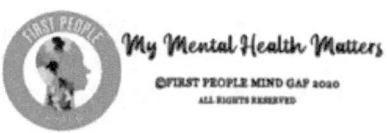

What makes a person think that they know what they are created to become from the plans of their creator is vision. See it, hear it, and walk into it to become it.

WHEN THE MIND SAY GO

BY MEISHA MERISHA

HEAD MIND AND LEGS
THE HEAD IS FULL
WHEN THE BODY SAYS GO
THE LEGS GETS WEAKEN BY THE KNEE
WHEN THE HEART SAYS GO
THE HANDS ARE SHAKEN LIKE A LEAF
BUT WHEN THE MIND SAYS GO
IS TIME TO STOMACH ALL AND MOVE

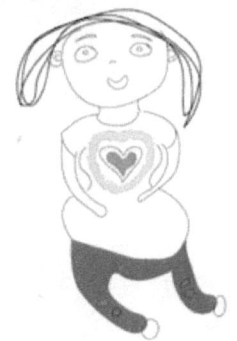

October 2013 Artist life performance

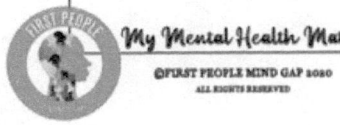

I did it. I couldn't believe I had made it, but I did it. In spite of the massive health challenge in my life that had been imposed on me, the enemy, I progressed and completed my therapeutic art diploma. This was a moment in my life when I walked around with a very heavy load on my body and mind – the load of a mental, emotional, open, unhealed wound from losing my brother suddenly as well as the load of physical bloat dropping down on my body, almost to the ground.

The poem is a caption of the story 'Then in a Nutshell', as it says, and what you see is what it was. I know now that although I was sometimes wavering with thoughts of suicide, even if I did not have the knowledge to acknowledge the presence of God, He was there all along, behind the scenes, waiting for me to see Him and invite Him in front of the screen.

◐ **Hair is the Glory** ◉

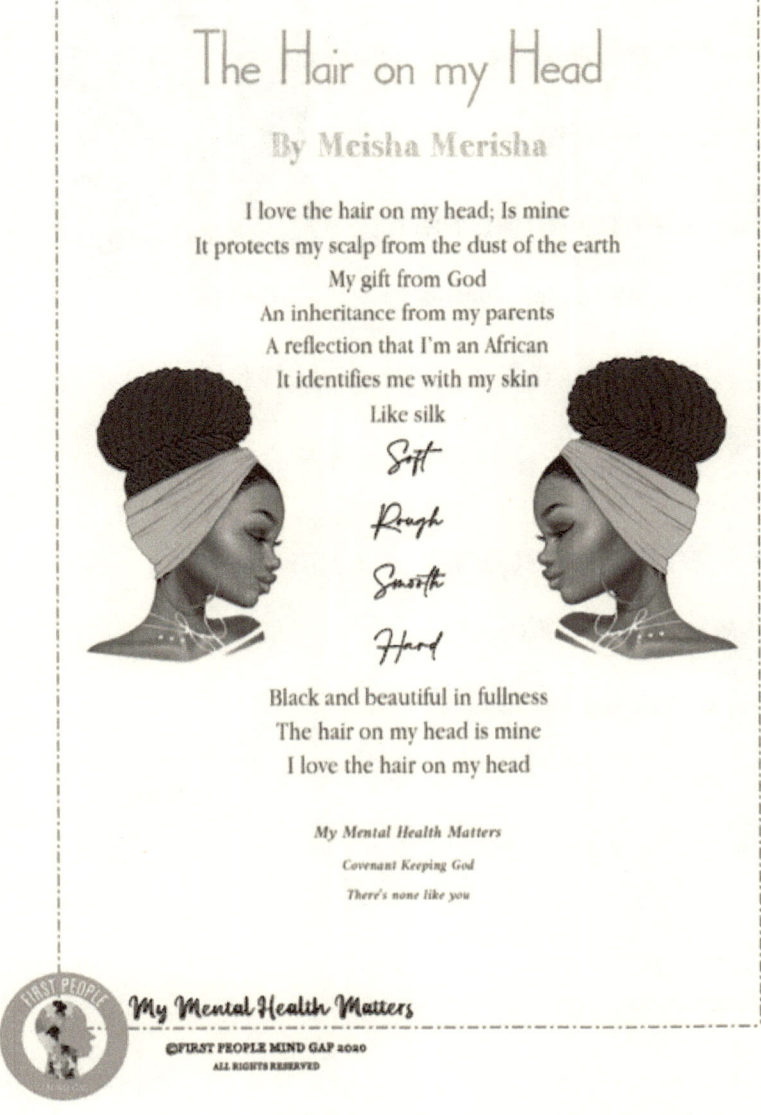

The Hair on my Head

By Meisha Merisha

I love the hair on my head; Is mine
It protects my scalp from the dust of the earth
My gift from God
An inheritance from my parents
A reflection that I'm an African
It identifies me with my skin
Like silk

Soft

Rough

Smooth

Hard

Black and beautiful in fullness
The hair on my head is mine
I love the hair on my head

My Mental Health Matters

Covenant Keeping God

There's none like you

My Mental Health Matters

The beauty of a woman is in her hair. Like the Bible says, the long length of a woman's hair is her glory.

FRIENDSHIP

F RIENDS STICK TOGETHER LIKE GLUE

R ESPECTFUL AND LOYAL

I NSPIRE YOUR FRIENDS

E NYOY THE GOOD TIMES TOGETHER

N EVER STOP BEING LOYAL AND KIND TO EACH OTHER

D ETERMINED AND EAGER LIKE A BEAVER TO HELP

S OMETIMES YOU FALL OUT BUT YOU GET BACK TOGETHER

H AVE CARE FOR EACH OTHER LIKE A MOTHER

I NTELLIGENT AND RELIABLE

P LEASING LIKE THE SUNSHINE

By Savannah Dos Santos
(Published in young writers London)

◯ Friendship ⊕

Friends are hard to find, so be careful. There are some people in our circle of friendship who are enemies, so we should be careful and know that it is better to be with one great friend than a thousand frenemies who are our rivals. Some of these people allow themselves to be used by the devil to wind up the days of their fellows in a negative direction so

190

that they can make wrong turns in life that would land them in a ditch off the road or, the worst case scenario, untimely death.

An explanation is given in the paperback *Compact Oxford English Dictionary*: 'A friend is a person that one likes and knows well, a person who supports a particular cause or organisation'. In the online dictionary, the definition of 'friend' is said to be 'a person with whom one has a bond of mutual affection, typically exclusive of sexual or family relations'. Friendship is a gift from God, so we should choose our friends with the view that we would fulfil one another; otherwise, it becomes forfeit.

Chapter V

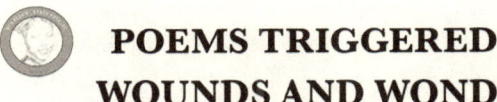

POEMS TRIGGERED BY WOUNDS AND WONDERS

By Merisha Meisha

Poems from the Heart

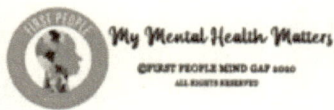

Poems from the heart, triggered up by wounds and wonders of life
By Meisha Merisha

May the real MR President Please Stand up!
Good day, good day,
Now that I got your attention;
Mr. President,
STEP ASIDE, DON'T STEP ON STAGE
Get in touch, put the light on
We have a right, keep your rice
Destinies are being destroyed, so stop saying it is well' with our money in your well!
Now that we got talking for a brief second'
Its good to hear your voice, allow us to speak with our own voice
One more thing!
When you take off in your private jet and you see the stars rising don't shut them down
to dust
Lastly. Listen very carefully to what every one of the people is saying now:
Don't cut our hair with the blade and make us look like slaves from the blazes. We are
real citizens of this land , and our birth rights from God has to be restored

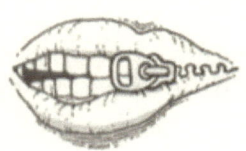

Melanin
Everything about me tells me everything
about myself
My hair
Nose
Lips
Hips
Bum
Bold, beautiful and bountiful

Stardust
Once upon a time,
The stars were dying rapidly and the sky
erupted tragically.
Darkness came and mysteriously,
something changed in the atmosphere.
Creating situations that can occasionally
make sporadic revelations.
When suddenly, affirmations of the
clouds appeared in the space that
disappeared into space.

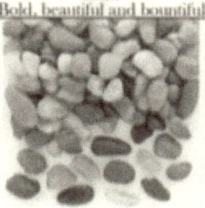

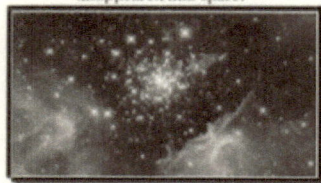

194

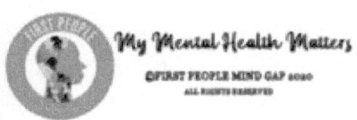

Wish upon the clouds

Don't think about dying for it may just come and kill you'
Just think about living, if you are still living'
Most people think of the day they are living'
Some people think of the day they've lived'
Live for the day you are living'
Stay in the day you are living'
And think about the day you are living in'
Don't think about dying, for it may just come and kill you because you're thinking
about dying instead of living
Think about living, and you will find that you are living

Death

Swiper, wiper, snapper, whippersnapper! Ugly sweeper!
You life taker and giver of none!
You turn off the lights of the living and take away their breath.
You came and you stole, and you took and you seized, what you've not been given.

You left me empty when you took my stars, and hid it in the well at Egunlane
You walked away with my right to have a family, when you swiped away my blood
brother off his feet.

Too tough to handle I jumped with my foot sinking in the soil
You pushed me high over the windows; I broke my leg like Jack
Unlike Jill I never recovered but slipped in deeper depth in debt
I slept deeper into death and never woke in-between the gap when I fell
You eliminated my face, exiled my mind and deposited his body by the train track for
your exchange in power.

You obliterate my life just to give you the euphoric efface gain and satisfaction to take
my place and gain power.

You are a bastard; you made me cry inside in silent, I could not even see my tears.

I was afraid to speak about how you snatched myself from from me, I remained in
silence and poured into a basket until I realized I was wasting away but could not get
away from the waste pit where you dumped my soul to sink in with the soil.

You nibbled as quickly as you swiped, and wiped when you stole my soul
You left me for death beneath my breath so I looked forward to the death that you laid
on me!

On a bright summer morning in middle of July, you chained me naked on the grounds
of a floor in a room under and tied my hands under the bed, in a place I no longer
recognize.

But a place where I met with the death that stole my soul and left me for dead, to face,
and smell the dying bloody blood of the dead.

You've never pleased the souls you captured in your cave
But yet trying to convince them that they rest better in a tunnel full of dark shades
Crowded in with black clouds in a gray sky' a thousand feet underneath
You hide your face in turmoil behind the soils in an empty box with no body in the
box; not even the bones of the bodies you took in the dark, you dirty liar.

Astonished are the folks who look down in despair under the grounds for what lays
below but have risen above.
Captivated are the souls of angles who are lifted unto the sky' opening with dazzling
sparks of lights. With a glaring shin as bright as the heaven where their soul rests in
peace' I hear an angel whispering into my very own soul; stay with me in your heart.
May our days be far with death not stealing you away from the sun like a thief at night
the way it came at me in a swipe at once in June., that ugly sweeper that stole my soul
away from the soils and brought me back to the dust before my time to be dusted off
before dawn, it was done and can't be undone.

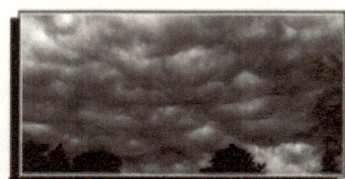

Men

Men are the starters of trouble
Men are the starters of trouble
They don't wash their hair
They don't clean their feet
They don't scrub their back
Men are the starters of trouble
Men are the starters of trouble
They don't wash their teeth
They use smelly shampoo
They have stinky feet
Men are the starters of trouble

Whole Me

I may not be the perfect baby
I may not be the perfect child
I may not be the perfect daughter
I may not be the perfect sister
I may not be the perfect niece
I may not be the perfect girlfriend
I may not be the perfect aunty
I may not be the perfect wife
I may not the perfect mother
I may not be the perfect grandmother as it
is in a man's eyes; I may be imperfect with
my conducts. But in God's eyes I'm the
perfect being working towards perfection
of my whole being.

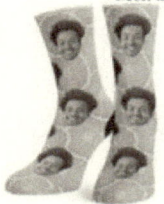

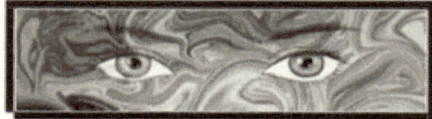

196

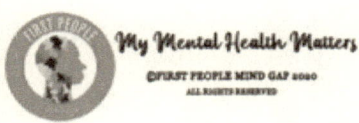

Legend

You're a legend for you gave, and you gave, and you kept giving

To be natured like you takes a man an extreme effort in growth to reach the levels of magnanimity that you've spread abundantly to all the babies you cradled in the family

The toddlers you backed that feed off your palms. You watched them fly as they spread their wings into the world; never failing to watch their backs even in their youths as they hopped on with their peers'

You watched the girls become ladies and saw the ladies become women as they learnt from the best and the best is you

In you the boys saw a legend, which you saw in them hero's, from youths a hero that grew form boys to men; men with extraordinary potentials and the accreditation to rule the world with the fear of God in their mind.

Mothers of all the children that you cared for once are now saying the children you cared for are now men, women, fathers and mothers of their own.

You would live in their hearts forever but in the hearts of their families will you remain also.

As I reserve a very special place in my heart for you, I only hope I live and experience that family solidarity that you've always wished upon the families that you touched with your love.

Angel of God, you remain a legend for I now know you were truly sent to earth for a reason and now that you've delivered whole heatedly your resting in the hands of our heavenly father, rest as we continue to miss you intensely.

Away from my body

Away from my body, I keep running as my soul gets berried into the soil
I smell the earth and feel the sea blowing on my left eye
I clinch unto the air whistling and wrestling with the hope to live one more day
I can feel my legs running into my belly but I walk without stretching a muscle
I run away from my body but a gust of wind swings my head to the right
I catch a glimpse of my footprints on the hot red sand in front of me
I continue to run forward without lifting a foot off the ground
I'm lifted off the floor' at the speed of the wind I cannot see
I spread my arms wide into the air
I swallow the waters and could taste the salt pouring into my mouth
I land at the edge of the shaw, and kept trying to sit up straight
I see my arms floating backwards but my feet keeps on flapping
I catch myself embracing the rocks that tied my legs deep in the sea
I can hear the wind blowing my chest back into the sea
I take a look at my body, my belly have disappeared from my body
I'm tankful for how far I've come this close to my body without a muscle
I stood up and walked away screaming' I'm free!

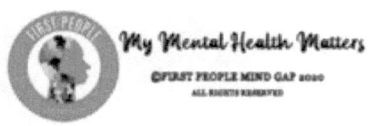

Lord who do you say I am
I am who I am
I am who I say I am
I am me'
I am, I am, I am
I am sure I am me'
I am all that I am
I am me' of course, I am me, me of course
I am not your definition of me because I am me
I am me in God who made me
I am a god, in me is god
Strong and powerful and made whole with the sound mind of
God

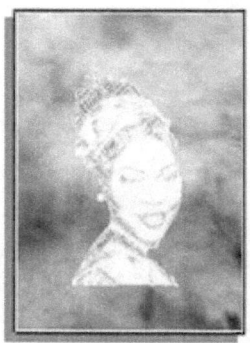

I Remember
I remember when I first saw you smile
I remember flying so high heights; I jumped high to fly higher when I saw a fly
I remember when I was a girl, I sat on a stool that broke into two with the woods on
each hand, I took and beat on a bucket that drummed so clamorously it travelled
forever until it landed on the emperor's head who sat on a stool that broke into two.

I remember when I walked alone thinking my mother was my invisible guardian angel.

I remember when I thought my grandpa was the god that protects my life over me.

I remember when I thought I could fly; like a fly.

I remember when I picked up a coin and gave it to a little old lady who backed a SON
on her back, and carried a basket on her head under the sun.

I remember singing in GRA. "NPN, Super Power. UPN, no Power". While my
neighbours sang. "UPN, Up! Up! Power. NPN, No Power!

I remember when I was a little girl, as modest as a pony; I danced in a room with rags
on the floor and a princess on a mat. Which made the princess take away her bow and
bowed for my dance.

I remember dancing in the rain with hails drops on my head just before I saw the
rainbow fizzle out with no trace on the clouds.

I remember stories I heard from the mouth of my mother's mother. She told them so
we knew we were the stories that we formed in our hearts,. So that we can tell our
children's children to hear the stories that made our mothers mother, the mothers of
the nation in our mother's land.

198

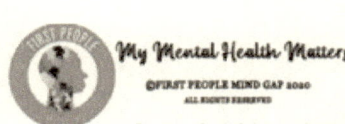

I remember sitting on hot white sand in the lands of Alidimma under a huge gwava tree that bears fruits so sour I bit my cheeks when trying to chew the seeds of the gwava that tasted so sour.

I remember I wrote in a dark wardrobe with delight' the stories of potato people in Sweden, of how they rolled on the grounds from pillar to post and eat each other on a piece of toast for dinner.

I remember MRS Jackie killed the children for tea and kept them in dark lakes for Jack to bake pasta for mama and papa.

I remember my skin burning under the sun on top of the mango tree
I remember the mangos falling from the mango tree when I sat under the tree
I remember seeing a snake fall from the mango tree that I sat under
I remember cutting my finger with a knife when I tried cutting a pawpaw
I remember crying behind the sofa because I did not want to go to the hospital to have my fingers stitched up. So I ran to catechism classes instead but the sister called my guardian, and my guardian said put that girl outside until I return, but never did come back.

I remember having a doll that cried a loud like a real baby but was taken away from me and never returned.

I remember seeing a magician stealing a boy from the crowd and he laid him for dead on the mat in front of the market square in town; which he laid on the floor for the coopers to tip him a copper or two so that he can wake the boy up who he laid for dead on the mat.
I remember telling my sibling the story of the boy who lay dead on the mat by the magician, and she said to me, 'Never ever stop to look at such things in your life so you don't disappear and never come home!

I remember my first valentine card so craftily made by hands it sent shivers to my livers that tickled me with joy because I never thought a boy would craft so carefully to win my heart by the be so crafty works of his hands.

I remember doing a daring thing when I ran after my older siblings to the river for the fun of it, knowing I can't swim. Suddenly I found myself in the deep ends of the river and I remember thinking I wish I could run back home with my legs across the river.

I remember thinking I'm sugar girl when I could neither read nor write, so I climbed on a chair I and washed the dishes that were pilled on the sink but did not stink in the sink.

I remember taking the meat from the pot of my neighbour's house, and how badly punished I was for this when the bowl of pepper I grained was inserted inside my fanny. This was not funny and made me wish on a bone to die because even the dogs were treated with more dignity than I.

I remember bathing with the boys from a bucket we all shared until I was told that girls should bath separately from boys.

I remember being scared walk in the dark without any lights.

I remember the thinking that I'm sitting on the toilet until I wet the mat and then realize bed-wetting.

I remember having a boyfriend when I did not even know the difference between a boy and a girl.

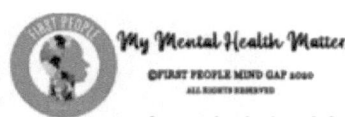

I remember having a lady maid that loved to be a lady, male driver that loved the car more than he loved to drive and a gate man that had a cane that smelt of blood.

I remember being beaten up at school in a fight with an older girl, I thought oh my god she's going to kill me.

I remember carrying a bucket of water on my head and being too careful not to let a drop of water fall out from the floor; I came back home with an empty bucket.

I remember playing with Jackie the dog that liked to jump on the bed, but ran away playfully until he was stolen.

I remember climbing on a stone to climb on a fence to climb on a tree pluck cashews just to get the cashew nut.

I remember thinking that there's skeletons down the pit toilet waiting to suck people down the hole.

I remember my sandals melting in the sun and then running with bear toes on hot sand

I remember the first time I fell in love with myself in front of the mirror

I remember thinking Anini is a rubber
I remember picking sails for stew from the garden
I remember eating ice cubes in the heat
I remember thinking little clever of me
I remember my first kiss was on the cheek
I remember holding hands with a boy to dump the bin
I remember watering my plants until they grew into a tree
I remember enjoying going to school
I remember you and me.

My Father's Face
Handsome and strong, behind his smile is a laugh clashing with his commands.
Oh what delightful joy it would be to see the smile hidden behind the structured figure reflect on my father's face.

In my Father's House
In my father's house there are many boys and girls
In my father's house
In my father's house
In my father's house there are many boys and girls
In my father's house, we fought for treats and attention most times
In my father's house we were excited, sad, angry, and sometimes hungry as can be!
But we were happy, happy, happy' as can be!
We were happy, happy, happy' as can be!

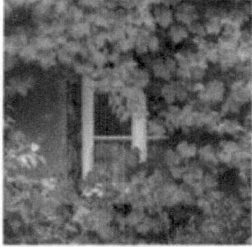

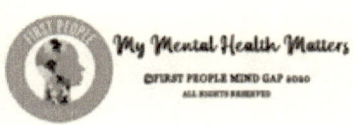

If Good is Bad

Bad is Good if good is bad. So if staying bad is good why do I itch so much to remain good.
While staying good is good why does it hurt so much to remain good And win in the battle of being bad I'm I good!

Solitude Misery

"Say hello to joy".
Happy said to sadness.

"Lets paint a picture for sadness".
Lonely whispered to happy with a sad face on his face but a painted happy face on his painting.

"Peep into happiness -".
Happy mutter standing tall with crossed hands.

"I do just well by myself".
Snapped sadness.

"Peep into happiness when it becomes dark inside and don't forget to leave lonely behind-". Happy said to sadness.

"I see you do just well inside all that aching and hurting because of
LONELINGNESS-".
Interrupted Misery with a defiant look on her face.

"Claim down! Shssh... now slowly, very, very slowly, slowly take a deep breath in and out and forget about lonely".
Happy said to sadness in a very low voice.

"Now wait on this rock for joy to pick up a peg before giving you a peck to peck you up".

"Woo! What great joy it is to be in the same shoes as happy".
Exclaimed sadness.

"You're very welcome to remain in my shoes".
Remarked happy with jazzy hands as he collapsed on mystery's shoulders shoving dejection off to land on its bottom.

"But it would be so unpleasant when lonely comes for tea to tease".

"I know; that's why you must keep a happy shoe on and remind lonely that you're better off dancing when alone.

MERISHA MEISHA

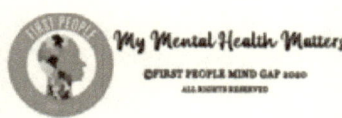

Connecting with myself

I'm a dog that I don't know when it's wanted

Is it that I sit on green grass chasing my tail until I know when I'm neglected and feeling dejected?

Or is it an illusion of fantasy that I'm rejected when in despair of dejection

Do I know when to be alone with sadness and joys of life, but shadowed with death and a glimmer of hope for life that I don't meet my death in the doom of death

Is it that I swim through the rivers under the tunnel for a peak of light in the day, with night drawing closer as I see the sparkles of the night resting on the flesh of my chest?

My Born Day

Thank you Lord for this day. Many years back' you blessed my parents with a beautiful baby.

They both welcomed me into their home and agreed that thereon I would be called the name they named men, and hoped my arrival would bring peace into the home.

The journey of my life began when I walk up my way of life with the touch light given to me from my father in heaven, and with the love shown to me by guidance on earth.

As bold as brass, I took sometimes gentle steps and other times wild jumps to hop over the hoops and holes in life.

Being careful not to avoid life in itself, but embracing life, as it is mostly bitter but especially beautiful.

I still remember to hold onto the light and love shown to me by my heavenly father.

Today that little person as it was a few years back is now enthroned in a new Kingdom. I've been entrusted in to serve as a servant of God, and by the grace' I identify myself now as a spiritual warrior guided light to do exploit in this Kingdom of God, not '**might**' but the grace of God; I'm happy to be in the Kingdom of God.

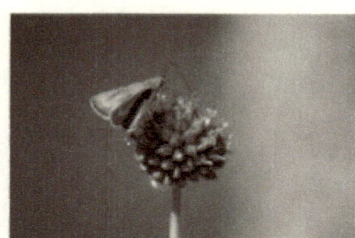

202

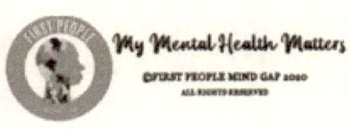

Mind Race

I'm running a race as fast as I can go even when my legs trip me, the faster I get.

The faster I run; the slower I become when falling becomes the greatest trick on track.

As rolling to the finish line proves effortless without moving a foot in front of the other,
I find myself rolling to the top but sliding back down only to realize that I was never at
the top!

So why take off at such a high speed in a rush only to get back at the top and realize that
I never once lifted a foot in front of the other to get to the top only to fall down to get
back up again right through to the top.

Behind the Stars

At first I wanted to reach for the stars
But bulrushes shiver's waters down my spine
While the ghost awaits a distant stare to share sprits
I witness the adorable silent; I dance with my words in a peaceful glee
And perceive the field of flowers kissed by the rain, yet before the crackle
The sandy storm blows a storm that clutters my mind with earthly worms
Still the candle burns but brighter for the languid shadows
The valley was lit with luminescence atmosphere
Nevertheless I lay struck with leaden weight from my life
Yet, I go to sea with a pod of peas in sack on my back
Spooky bloody red velvet desert gushing down the fountain on a mountain of ice
In the hospitality of when I go high and low searching'
Howbeit I'll never know the secrets behind the stars
Until it's reveled by the shadows within the stars

Feeling Me Feel me

I cry not because I'm weak but because I'm in touch with my feelings
I speak out not because I'm rude but because I'm direct
I challenge what I hear not because I'm confrontational but because I'm opinionated
I make my decisions not because I'm stubborn but because I know my choices
I ask not because I'm inquisitive only, but because I care
I love not because I'm needy but because I've a heart
I'm confidence not because I'm arrogant but because I've God's Grace
I'm genuine to myself not because I'm proud but be I'm unique
I'm wired not because I'm a wiredo but because I'm created with peculiar gifting's
I'm blessed not because I've money but because I'm rich in the glory of God.

203

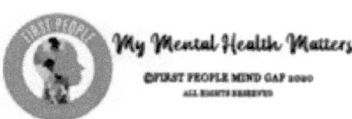

After the rain comes the sunshine

After the rain comes the sunshine
By the time I realise myself, I hope it's not too late
But there's nothing hidden under the sun
Under the sun
Under the sun
The creator of the moon stars and sun knows all the secrets on the cloud
I'm not a clown to think I know better than He who knows me even before I was
formed in the womb
Now he found me under the rocks and placed me on the rock even with the shield and
the spells
I see after the rain comes the sunshine for me to shine before it's too late

The Word

Hear it
Think it
See it
Believe it
Say it
Have it as the word says it.

MY MENTAL HEALTH MATTERS

Chapter VI

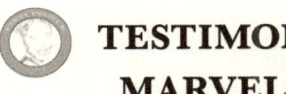 **TESTIMONIES OF GOD'S MARVELLOUS WORKS**

Testimonies

There's power in the special blood of Jesus Christ. I am sharing a few of these testimonies with you so that God will also grant you, your friends, and your family supernatural healing and turn tests into testimonies with speed.

My prayer for you is that God will replicate these miracles and reveal His marvellous self to you as you lean on Him for guidance and assurance. I also pray that as you search for the joy of the Lord, His joy will fill up that void in your heart so that your joy will always be renewed into rejoicing until the perfect day of Jesus's return in His mighty name.

I am also sharing my testimonies with you because I have vowed to return all the glory to God almighty, who has given me multiple buckets of testimonies for me to testify His goodness in my life, thereby making my life a testimonial. He alone should be glorified in the mighty name of Jesus Christ.

> 'The man who saw it has given testimony, and his testimony is true. He knows that he tells the truth, and he testifies so that you also may believe.'

> **—John 19:35 (New International Bible)**

◔ February 2021 ◑

February 2021: Exam Success — Ms Sandra S., West London

Good morning, Merisha. Thank you for messaging. I have been thankful to the Lord; He helped me pass that paper I have not been able to pass since 2018! PRAISE JESUS! The exam didn't go as well as I hoped, but I still managed to pass, and it's all to the glory of God.

I used your 'pray to God like it's already yours' advice, and my heavenly Father really came through! I am so happy and so blessed! It's like a miracle based on how I passed. God hasn't forgotten me; He's making me mentally stronger day by day. I can see that God is so powerful, and henceforth, I have been so grateful to Christ Jesus recently.

◔ September 2019 ◑

September 2019: Mental Health Sanction Cancelled — Ms Joy, Princess Royal University Hospital, Orpington, Kent

I received the news that a sister of mine had been admitted into the hospital with regard to her ill mental health. I found the news troublesome because of the nature of the illness and the reoccurrence of admission into the mental health hospital. I am privileged to be a sanctuary keeper by the Lord's direction at my place of worship. On a faithful Sunday, after service, we held a sanctuary keepers' meeting. In this meeting, I was sitting next to a sister called Joy who coincidentally bears the name of the sister I was going to visit at the hospital, but I know with God, there are no coincidence, so I promised God that I would return to share my testimony as soon as He showed me what to do.

I believed that God had led me to sit next to Joy as a sign to show me that He had heard my prayers because this was the first time I was seeing Joy, and I was going to see my sister Joy at the hospital that same Sunday after service. As I could sense there was a connection with Joy in my spirit, I confided in her, and we had a prayer of agreement so that on my arrival at the hospital, I would meet Joy with a sound spirit.

On my arriving at the hospital, Joy told me that she had been sanctioned under the mental act for three months and that as a result of this, her mood was plummeting, and she feared the responsibilities that awaited her. I did not have any of the answers to the questions that she had asked me, but I knew someone who had all the answers. So I prayed over a mantle, but before handing her the mantle, I took us into some scriptures to enhance our understanding of the mystery of the mantle. I also declared that she would be discharged within three weeks and not up to three months. To the glory of God, she had a hearing within two weeks of my visitation; in the hearing, she was told that the sanction had been removed and that she was free to reunite with her family.

There is an awesome power in the mystery of the mantle; just like Elijah passed on his mantle to Elisha, so does this power flow in the midst of the Winners Chapel family, from the bishop David Oyedepo down to his spiritual children.

'And it came to pass, when they were gone over, that Elijah said unto Elisha, "Ask what I shall do for thee before I be taken away from thee." And Elisha said, "I pray thee, let a double portion of thy spirit be upon me."'

— 2 Kings 2:9

◐ August 2019 ◉

August 2019: Settlement — Mrs Ellie G. A., South London

I met Merisha in South East London when I newly arrived from Sweden to join my husband in London. At the time of our meeting, I was looking for a job and looking for channels on how best to integrate into the London lifestyle. So meeting Merisha was a really good icebreaker as she was very open with sharing her knowledge with me about London and how to secure a job interview. I found Merisha's instructions very useful as I soon got a job offer to work with the Council on Transport for Disabled Students.

Some years later, I wanted to change my job for a job that was flexible for me to manage working and looking after my children. I called Merisha, and I was surprised at how quickly she had connected me directly with my next job (working with families), which provided a lot of flexibility for me.

Over the years, I have found Merisha trustworthy because I know she's a woman of God, and this brings me to have confidence in confiding in her. There was a time I experienced delays in receiving my British passport. I called Merisha and said I wanted her to pray with me about the delays. She prayed with me without any hesitation and committed the matter to God. In the wake of her prayer and less than three months following her praying with me on the matter, my British passport was released.

I remember the day I called Merisha to share this testimony with her; she told me that she was just about to walk into a midweek service, which is at the Winners Chapel in Dartford, Kent, but she said something that was intriguing: 'I know they have released your passport. Praise God.'

I was and still am intrigued by the confidence Merisha had that God would definitely grant our request in prayers for my status to change. I truly am grateful to God, who answers prayers, and I give Him all the thanks and reverence.

◯ April 2019 ◉

April 2019: Toothache Healed and Dental Surgery Cancelled — Abdul S., East London

God healed my Muslim boss from severe toothache in April 2019. This healing took place very shortly after I joined Abdul's organisation as a healthcare coordinator. Abdul, who was my direct manager at the time of the healing, had exclaimed that the pain he felt was excruciating. He also explained that the pain was the result of a terrible toothache coming from the lower part of his mouth.

On the day the healing occurred, Abdul was clearly in distress. He paced in and out of the office. I could hear him making over the phone an emergency dental appointment at 1600 hours that same day. This appointment had already been made by him after his dental surgery, which saw the removal of some of his teeth, but the purpose of this call was to advance the dated appointment as his faith was tied down by the performance of the dentist operating on his mouth.

While he was looking for an assistant to drive him to the dentist, I was thinking that the only solution I could offer to resolve his issue was to offer him prayer and trust in God to do the healing. However, while this inspiration was passing through my mind, another thought was also rushing through my head: 'Who do I think I am to pray for my Muslim boss?' I too was, at the time, experiencing a toothache that lasted for a year exactly.

However, as Abdul's ordeal was prolonged, I could no longer bear hearing him say, 'I am dying. I have to pull my tooth out!' I felt increasingly uncomfortable hearing him exclaim this in agony, so I plucked up the courage and encouraged myself to talk with him. Even though Satan was using the fact that I had a toothache to drum doubt into my mind that he would not be cured, I stood on the truth that Jesus Christ, the Son of God who died on the cross of Calvary, would heal him because I was trusting God with the healing of my boss, and so I held on to this faith.

Moving on, I did not want any other person's interference to contaminate our discussion, so I excused us from the office, and we sat on the seats against the walls by the corridor's hallway landing of the tall building. Here, I told Abdul that if he accepted that I was going to pray for him in the name of Jesus, it was God that would heal him in that name of Jesus Christ the King. To my astonishment, he accepted.

I prayed a prayer that lasted for less than a minute, but I remembered to recite this prayer with thanksgiving as I had been taught by my bishop, David O. Oyedepo. This prayer consisted of thanksgiving in the beginning, middle, and end. I then brought out from my bag a very small portion of anointing oil and the Holy Communion and shared it with Abdul.

The next day, when Abdul returned to work, he began to call me a healer. He went round to the other departments of the company in other parts of town announcing that I am a healer. By now, I already know through learning the word of God that my soul would be in jeopardy should I contemplate on stealing the work of the Holy Spirit functioning through me. Now as genuine as it may seem for Abdul to call me a healer based on this theory, he may not be aware of the spiritual rules concerning who to give reverence to when the function of God's work is pronounced in a man's life.

I already knew it was the Holy Spirit that was quick at work to distinguish me in my workplace. Again, I know already that I cannot claim God's work no matter the position or fame that awaits me. It would have been foolishness for me to keep my mouth closed at a time when I should say it is the Lord's doing and it is marvellous in the eyes of men. My reaction was only based on the obedience of following the lead of the Holy Spirit so as to see His works manifest through me.

I quickly corrected Abdul that Yeshua, who is Jesus Christ, was the doer of the works and the one who healed the tooth in his mouth; I was just a vessel that God used to perform the miracle – similar to the pipe that carries water from the tap onto the tank, which does not mean that the pipe is producing the water because the water is coming from the ground. I wasn't permitted to receive thanks for the works of God because all the glory must return to Him so that He can continue to remain with me while performing miracles through me, like He did for Saint Paul in **Acts 19:11**.

Abdul was puzzled with my response and was insisting on the fact that I had some healing powers. He said that if he was not allowed to call me a healer, he should call me a doctor instead. Rather than allow his praise to get to my head, I enlightened him with Jeremiah's inspiration: 'Is there no balm in Gilead; is there no physician there? Why then is not the health of the daughter of my people recovered? (**Jeremiah 8:22**)'

By engaging Abdul in a way of understanding the power in the name of Jesus Christ, I believe my faith also increased because I suddenly noticed that my own toothache was healed, and for the first time in a year, I began to chew with the affected tooth. I could now bite on the tooth where the dentist wrongly diagnosed me and performed an irrational dental procedure in 2018 when I went in to report symptoms of a toothache.

It takes just a little faith to believe what great things God can do, and to my greatest amazement, in an environment where I was feeling unsure, God showed me what a humorous God He is because he showed up on my behalf and reassured me that He is in me all the time so that I can confidently declare that He who is in me is greater than he who is in the world, as described in **Deuteronomy 31:6**: **'Be strong and courageous. Do not fear or be in dread of them, for it is the Lord your God who goes with you. He will not leave you or forsake you.'**

All I have to do is believe and trust God, knowing that He is too faithful to fail me and that fear will diminish because the greater the faith, the smaller the fear. Even if fear is a reoccurrence with life challenges as it is the carrier of doubt, know that believing in what God can do is also the channel to magnify your miracle as faith is the reassurance that you will overcome the challenges that you face.

In the same week, Abdul said that he would look into creating a prayer room in the workplace so that it was available when needed. This goes to show that Jesus Christ is the master physician who is always at work. To this point, when you activate your awareness of this truth, you will see fireworks from the hands of the Father. Hallelujah to the LORD almighty; to Elohim be all the glory!

June 2018

June 2018: Divine Intervention; Lungs Healing — Mr Martins, Queen Elizabeth Hospital, South East London

On a Wednesday, at midday, before visiting the hospital, I prayed that God would remove people who positioned themselves on the streets as an opposition to obstruct the work of God in people's lives and as an obstacle to prevent people from receiving the gospel.

At first, when I left my house, I had no idea of what direction I should head into; I just knew I had to head out and tell somebody that they were loved by God almighty. I did ask the Holy Ghost to lead me to where I ought to be so that the people He wanted me to reach would be the first to partake of receiving the good news of the love of Jesus Christ and accepting the Saviour into their lives.

Shortly after leaving home, I found myself at my local bus stop. I began a conversation with a man I met for the first time through sharing a testimony with him about a time when God favoured me. Yes, there have been several times when God has shown me His mercy and favour, as He does for you as well, but there is one element to recognising God's favour in our lives, and there is another element to testifying God's favour in our lives. ***A testimony that is testified is one that is intensified.***

As my testimony unravelled, it extended into a dialogue because of the inquisitive attitude of the man; questions poured out in the case of our prolonged conversation, and we exchanged thoughts on the fruitfulness of God's faithfulness. I ended up at the hospital stop eventually. I interrupted the flow of our conversation because I had my mind made up that I would hop off at the hospital stop, where I would share the good news of the love of God to the people starting from the entrance of the hospital.

When I arrived at the hospital, I thanked God for ordering my footsteps because it was only upon my arrival at the hospital that I recalled previous prompting by the Holy Spirit to volunteer my time in kingdom services at the hospital, praying for people to receive salvation and to be healed. I saw a group of people smoking; some were standing round others who were sitting on the bench, but one person was sitting on a wheelchair. So I walked towards then, and after exchanging greetings with them, I began to share my testimony with the people about the time in 2016 when the Holy Ghost took away my smoking habit from me in a very profound way.

Almost shortly after I had begun to speak to the people gathered, I noticed that they ceased their previous discussions and began to engage with the message that I was delivering to them. Ultimately, as the discussions progressed, there was a fierce woman emerging into the group. This strange woman refused to acknowledge my person or accept my message, and her aim was to scatter the meeting. However, before she could disperse the group, I managed to gain the attention of another woman who introduced me to a young man named Martin and nicknamed Marty.

Although I could sense that Martin was coated with fear when he called me aside and began to explain his predicament to me, his greater fear was uncertainty about an operation to be performed on his lungs. Aside from this, he confided in me that he did not have a phone to allow fluency for me to follow him up, even though he had his number on him. So I promised to arrive early at the hospital with a phone for him the following morning.

On my arrival at the hospital the following morning, I went to Martin's ward, but I was told that he had been transferred. As soon as I began to make enquires on where he had been transferred to, the same woman who had tried to dispose of me the day before came out unexpectedly and began to contend against the nurse's decision to tell me where Martin's new location was, and her claims were that I was a stranger to him. Thank God the nurse asked me who I was and I was given the opportunity to introduce myself as Martin's new friend. I told the nurse that Martin was the one who had given me both the invitation and permission to pray for him. After hearing what I had to say, the nurse did not hesitate to direct me to Martin's designated ward.

When I walked into the new ward at the hospital, the first person I saw working around the reception desk was one of my neighbours who lived only a few doors away from my house. I don't know how God arranged it this way so that my neighbour would see me at work for God. I later understood that it was because of what God was about to do so that men could see that He is my true living God, with His eyes all round me.

Unfortunately for the devil, who wanted to stop Martin from having an encounter with God, I met Martin still at the Queen Elizabeth Hospital in Woolwich. He waited anxiously at his bedside, waiting to be transferred yet again but this time to another hospital that was better equipped for the nature of his operation. Martin had no way of communicating with me prior to my arrival or believing that I would fulfil my promise of visiting him again, knowing that his location had been moved. Still, gladly, we met, and he was able to explain to me the development of his condition, which had elevated to critical.

Martin explained that an urgent scan had revealed the collapse of his lungs, and as a result of this change, the transfer team was in the process of taking him to the Charing Cross Hospital in Hammersmith for an emergency surgery because the Queen Elizabeth did not have the facilities for his operation. So he was being monitored before the ambulance team came to transfer him to the Charing Cross Hospital.

I felt very privileged to be appointed by God on behalf of Martin's aid. At the same time, I did not know how God was going to turn this situation around. All I knew was that I had to trust God in the process to perfect the performance of the operation. I could not be scared if I was the one who had been sent to pray for the one who lay scared on the hospital bed.

Driven by my spirit, I visited the hospital in the early hours of that morning, prepared with my anointing oil, the Holy Communion, a mantle, and the Winners Chapel Chronicle of Miracles. Before any of these mysteries were administered, I invited Martin to join me in the family of Jesus Christ through the salvation lane, and he willingly accepted. I brought out the Chronicle of Miracles and read some of the testimonies at the front to Martin. After this, I turned to the back and read the prayer of salvation aloud for Martin. He repeated after me so that the vows were openly confessed and were his to declare to the Lord God almighty. ***The word of God says that faith comes by hearing the wonders and works of God.***

◯ **Prayer of Salvation** ◉

'Lord Jesus, I come to you today. I am a sinner, but you died for me. Jesus, I invite you into my life. Be my Lord and Saviour and save me from a life of sin. Now I know that I am born again.'

Before I left Queen Elizabeth Hospital, I saw an orange juice bottle on the table that belonged to Martin. The bottle had a straw inside it, so I gave him the anointing oil to add to the juice if he felt comfortable doing that. I then gave him the Holy Communion and encouraged him to take the communion and the anointed juice if he believed in God for a miracle. I also left him a mantle as a gift and again committed him to God by requesting from God to do for Martin what I requested from Him for myself, and that was for God to heal Martin and allow the doctors to take care of him. I handed over the phone and charger to Martin, and then I left the building feeling lighter than when I had walked in. On reaching home that Thursday, I decided to dance in praise to the Lord in advance on behalf of Martin to thank God for healing him in advance.

On Friday, day three of my meeting with Martin, I went to Brixton in South London for a very important meeting. On my return, while I was waiting at the train station, my phone rang. It was Martin ringing. He called to let me know that he had been transferred successfully to the Charing Cross Hospital as proposed, but upon arrival, he was examined; all the tubes that had been inserted into his body for investigation were removed, and he was sent home.

He said, in his very own words, **'I am just calling to let you know that I have just gotten the all-clear and I have been discharged home.'**

There was a pause.

'I don't know what happened, but as soon as they took off the tubes, the pain disappeared.'

I replied, telling him, 'God happened.'

Then he said, 'Yes. I'm coming to serve your God.'

The woman who introduced me to Martin on the day I met them all sitting outside also called me and was in tears of joy, saying, almost singing, the following: **'I know of what God can do. This is why I wanted you to talk with Martin. Since I have known him all these years, he has never been to any church, but for the first time in his life, he took himself to church to give thanks to God, and this made me cry.'**

I said, 'Praise God almighty.'

I shared this testimony on the pulpit, but I could not elaborate on all the components of the testimony in sixty seconds. Having said that, I captured as much as I could in a minute. After I stepped down from the pulpit, a few people congratulated me for my testimony, while others thanked me for sharing such an inspiring testimony. My reply to all was that I thanked God, and I also congratulated them in advance as I too was looking forward to hearing their own testimonies of when they went to heal the sick in the name of Jesus Christ.

Consequently, while I was in the midst of the congratulations, a mummy whom I was familiar with and who was known to be always joyous to all, approached me and said, **'I heard your testimony. I am so jealous.'**

Should I believe that she was truly jealous, or was she joking? 'Why joke with venom on one's tongue?' I wondered, but as it goes, to this date, I noticed that she stopped regarding me or accepting my salutes since the day I shared my testimony. I noticed this behaviour, but I did not confront her or confirm it from her as this was not the first time I had seen people despair as my testimonies increased, people closer, even so in increasing numbers. However, this mummy's case was peculiar because she was vocal about her feelings of failing to absolve the fact that I had not done the works but only positioned myself in a location at times in my life when I allowed God to use me.

I also do not underestimate the mysterious works of God, so every testimony of the wonderful acts of God in my life gets me ecstatic and still alarms me no matter how many ages back the miracle had been performed to add to my experience of Christ. If the Holy Spirit is eminent in me, it's because I magnify His works in my heart and then testify this to the world with my being no matter how trivial people may think the event is. There is no small testimony in my book, especially after hearing Pastor Nathaniel Odain comment, **'No testimony of God is embarrassing.'**

After that, I testified about my freedom from masturbation on the pulpit. The full narration of this corporeal escape has been documented and imprinted onto my electronic journal.

The woman whom God will use is one who would place her heart in a fragment that would allow the Holy Spirit to penetrate her mind.

◐ July 2017 ◉

July 2017: Professional Football Career Restored and Family Reunion — Alberto N., England

'I testify to the Lord. Over a week ago, I was encountering some serious problems with my finances and career. This made things very difficult for me. Before I travelled during the holidays, I met Merisha when she was evangelising in South East London by the Royal Woolwich Arsenal Station. She gave me her number and invited me to attend a Sunday service, but I wasn't able to attend because I was due to travel. However, while I was travelling, the club that I played football for called me to inform me that they had released me from their club.

'In the midst of these challenges that I suddenly found myself in, I began to feel the pain from being released from my club, and all the problems that were piling on me unsettled me. So I sent Merisha a text message at two o'clock in the morning – just as well because I could not sleep – and my text read, **'Pray for me.'**

'Although Merisha never knew who it was at the time, she called me back to find out who it was that could be texting at such hours in the morning. I could hear from her voice that she was concerned because of the nature of my text message. I explained to Merisha how she had met me at the Royal Arsenal Woolwich Station while she was evangelising some months back. Merisha asked me if I was OK first, and then she prayed for me, but before she began to pray for me, she asked me if I believed in God. I said yes, and then she told me to believe that it was God who would perform the miracle I was expecting.

'The Sunday following my call, Merisha invited me to church for the *Covenant Day of Supernatural Turnaround Sunday Service*. During the service, I heard a man of God, Pastor Nicolas Udoh, advising the congregation to pay attention to the service, connect with the service, and believe in what God would do as an after-mark of the service. Pastor Udoh then declared and decreed that two minutes past twelve o'clock tomorrow, Monday, someone here would have a supernatural turnaround. As soon as I heard this declaration proclaimed, I received this message in my heart as a word of prophecy and then found instant peace of mind. When I got back home from the service, I decided not to pick up any calls. I was unexplainably happy and found rest more in myself after I diverted all my incoming calls onto my voice mail. I then decided to go out jogging.

'The immediate Monday after the Sunday service, when I came back from my football practice in the morning, I noticed that someone I didn't know contacted me on Twitter. He told me that he worked on behalf of the FIFA football agent and that he had seen me play before but did not have the time to contact me because he was on a trip in London, but if I was interested, he would like to manage my football profession. He asked me to drop my number on his email, so I did and waited patiently for a response.

'Exactly two minutes past twelve o'clock, I received a call from the FIFA agent. He told me that he would like to discuss the terms of the contract with me, and if I was all right with it, they would let me know what the next step was. I agreed but informed him that he should be as clear and transparent with the contract as possible so that I knew what I was agreeing to. On Thursday, he called me and told me to forward my CV and passport to him. He told me to be expectant and that he would get back to me.

'On Saturday, while I was getting ready to attend the house fellowship meeting, I got a call from my auntie. She was not feeling so good, so I decided to go and see her. "Coincidentally", while I was at my auntie's place, I got the phone call from the agent, and he said that they had established the terms of the contract, and so they would like to give me the contract, even though I did not have the visa type that they required for me to be accepted on the team. God granted me a career breakthrough because the man of God had decreed the word of God that guided me in the course of the service.

'The agent directed me to the embassy with a referral letter that should grant me the visa required for me to go ahead with the rest of the team. As if this was not enough, miraculously, at that same hour of me receiving the call from the agent, my sister who had been missing from our home gatherings and had not maintained any contact with any member of the family returned home and walked through the door. Praise God!'

Although I could still hear Gilberto's testimony from the recording on my phone, I could hear the force of my voice vibrating in a scream; I shouted 'MY JESUS!' repeatedly as I went ballistic over Gilberto's testimony. After the service, I was given permission by Gilberto to record his full testimony, and this is what I have shared with you already. Even reading about it now in November 2020 in this book, it feels like this testimony was delivered only yesterday, and I can almost taste the JOY today. What's more is that in 2020, when I saw Gilberto, he was still going strong in his football career. Praise God!

I pray for you and your family that as you read the testimonies in this book, the Spirit of the LORD, Christ Yeshua, would transform your life though the mystery of the blood of the lamb and draw you into salvation as you submit your soul to Him, thereby making your life a testimonial in the mighty name of Jesus Christ. If you believe God can do this, say AMEN loudly. Read Gilberto's testimony printed in the Chronicle of Miracles at the time he testified the wonders of God's doing in his life:

'I am a professional footballer from Spain. I played with the second division club and was asked by an agent to come to London to play for the Tottenham Spurs. I cancelled my contract with the Spanish club and relocated to London in 2016, but when I got here, the agent abandoned me. I was stranded and had to resort to a lifestyle that was below the standard I was used to. I found work with a smaller club for less pay. I was depressed and dejected.

'A lady who attends this church invited me to attend one of the services, but I told her that I would call her when I returned from a planned holiday. While on holiday, I received a call from my current club that I had been released, and I was shocked and sad. I sent a text to the lady to pray for me as I thought my world was falling apart. This was at two o'clock in the morning. She prayed for me and led me to Christ. I came to church last Sunday, and the pastor prophesied there would be a supernatural breakthrough at twelve two the next day. He encouraged us, saying that since it was going to be a miracle, we only needed to believe.

'A man who said he works on behalf of a FIFA agent contacted me via Twitter and asked to be my manager as he had followed me for some time. He asked for my phone number, and the next day, at exactly 12:02 p.m., the FIFA Agent called me and said he had seen me play in London and wanted to manage me. By Thursday, he asked me to send copies of my CV and passport to him. That same day, my aunt called me, and we welcomed my sister whom we had not seen for five years back home. Thereafter, I received the call that my new contract had been confirmed. Praise the Lord!'

◐ April 2017 ◉

April 2017: Escaped Suicide Attempt via Divine Intervention — Rita, South East London

I met Rita at the lounge in the local council with three of her youngest children. I began talking with Rita and gave my number to her and then left it up to her to call me whenever she pleased.

A couple of weeks after our first encounter, I saw Rita looking helpless in front of a solicitor's office in Woolwich, South East London. I went to her and asked if she was OK. It was then that Rita opened up to me and told me that the social services team had removed her five children from her; she said that they had been rehoused because of certain issues, which were coupled with a conspiracy from her ex-partner in a fight to gain full custody over their children. Rita expressed that she felt down as a result of it and was waiting to see a lawyer who could take on the case.

However, on my arrival home, I received a text message from Rita, who wrote that she was on the verge of committing suicide. The text message read, **'I feel like killing myself. Without my children, I want to die.'**

I was slightly shocked based on my reasoning that Rita should see that the best was yet to come even though she was in a very tough situation. On the outside, I could somehow see a glorious end to her challenges. Still, my reasoning did not limit me from being empathetic towards her circumstances, so this left me concerned for Rita, but the only way I knew was to commit my sorrows to God.

I invited her to the Sunday service so that she could hear the word of God to lift up her spirits and renew her joy. During the service, during praise time, Rita was encouraged not to sit down crying but to get up and dance in praise to the Most High God almighty, the creator of the universe who sees the deep cut of her heart that no one else has access to.

The following Saturday, I invited Rita to the house fellowship group, which she went to alone. During testimony time, I was surprised when Rita shared her testimony: in the space of a week, the miracle-working power of God located her and rehoused her with a bigger apartment. As if that was not enough, she added that her five children had been brought back to her with 'apologies' for the disruption caused in her family.

I wish you yourself reading about this testimony now and smiling to yourself were present at the house fellowship to witness the awe on all of our faces as Rita shared her testimony. All stood aside in awesome wonder at the speed at which the almighty moved to terminate the frustration in Rita's life; because she came a little bit closer to Him, He took away her worries and gave her wonders.

I pray that the Most High God almighty take away your shame today and give you fame in that same area of concern, subtle fame so that the glory of God in your life will make you glow and grow globally for all to know that the one and only living God is on the go for good. Amen.

March 2017

March 2017: Divine Healing (Skin Infection) — Melanie, South East London

On a faithful day in March 2017, I was out on evangelist duties when I met Anthony at the entrance of Tesco in South East London. My conversation with Anthony kick-started when he greeted me familiarly as someone he already knew. Anthony is the father of Melanie, whom God healed. On our meeting, I took the opportunity to minister the word of God to him. After I ministered the word to him, Anthony expressed his major concern at that time to be his daughter's skin condition; she was covered in eczema, all over her body. Anthony told me that they were both unable to sleep at night and that most nights, they both stayed up scratching until the skin began to bleed on the bedding.

Surprisingly enough I actually got excited and angry at the same time when Anthony shared Melanie's health condition with me. (This feeling of excitement and holy anger comes upon me most times when I see my confidence in God increase. I am angry on one hand that the devil is afflicting people as a mission, but on the other hand, I am excited, knowing that the hands of God are sure to settle the matter quickly.)

Relating to my own experience, I was angry because the fourth night prior to meeting Anthony, I saw that a patch of eczema had sprung up on my belly all of a sudden. I know how irritating and discomforting it is to have an unpleasant itch on the skin, but I remember how God healed me supernaturally. So I was too excited already and overly interested in laying my prayers for Melanie to the one and only living God.

Before commencing my prayer though, I did ask Anthony if I could meet and pray for Melanie in a location they both felt comfortable with. Anthony invited me to their home and explained that Melanie had been traumatised by the experience of her skin condition; they had tried all the medical procedures and prescriptions since Melanie was a baby, all coming to nil or disproven to have worked in eradicating the problem.

I went to see Melanie with a tiny bottle of anointing oil, a small box of Holy Communion, and a single square piece of mantle cloth, which I presented to her as a gift from Jesus Christ. The night before I went to see Melanie, I prayed all night so that God would heal her and relieve her from the pain and sleepless nights instantly and so the whole wide world would know that it was His doing alone.

During my consultation with Anthony, Anthony restated that he and his family had been applying all sorts of medical cream on Melanie's skin but to no avail. So I encouraged him to put all the doctor's prescriptions aside for the moment and just apply the anointing oil on Melanie's skin. I also advised that other times, he should add the anointing oil to Melanie's orange juice and give her the communion to eat, but when she was going to bed, he should give her the mantle to take with her, like she did with her soft teddy.

I whispered to Melanie, **'Jesus Christ will be protecting you because He cares for you and loves you so much. He wants your skin to be beautiful like His.'**

I gave her the mantle and told her to take it to bed when she was going to sleep, just like she took her teddy bear with her, but this time, she would be taking her mantle with her so that Jesus Christ would protect her throughout the night. I spoke to Melanie as if the eczema on her skin was a thing of the past already. I spoke to her with faith on my mind and showed it with my eyes. I did not speak to her in baby talk but in a baby tone so that she could be keen to hear me. I trusted the Holy Ghost to bring her to the understanding that she needed to receive it in her young spirit, and then I left my conversation in the hands of the Most High God almighty to take care of our communion. Melanie nodded to indicate she had understood, and I hoped she had understood me too.

The next morning, I saw a missed call following a text message on my handset. The message was from Anthony, and it exclaimed that for the first time, father and daughter were able to sleep at night without any itching on the skin. So I called him back immediately, but it was little Melanie who answered the phone.

'Thank you, Aunty. That made my skin better' came her innocent voice.

'Jesus Christ made your skin better, not me.' This was my reply to her.

On 13 June 2017, I went to visit Melanie as a follow-up, and I did believe my eyes when I saw the beautiful works of my heavenly Father, but I admit I was reduced to tears of joy to see the reality of this answering prayer from God. I held my tears back but could not contain myself for long or wait until I got home to express myself solely to God. As soon as I got to the field round the corner from Anthony's house, I collapsed on the green fields and lifted my face to the sky, and tears of joy poured out in my appreciation to God for a quick, sharp miracle. I tried to stop myself from crying, but I carried on crying on my way home. I cried openly and praised God heartily for turning my tears of pain in hope that He would heal Melanie in no time to tears of joy in the twinkle of an eye.

Shortly after feeling a teardrop on my skin, I realised I had been crying. Amazed, I texted my then resident pastor Nicolas Udoh: 'I'm just returning from the house of the brother whose daughter I prayed for in April, and she received her healing. I SAW IT WITH MY EYES! My God is big and mighty. I'm full with tears of JOY!' What amazed me most was the way Melanie's skin healed with no scars or traces that she ever had eczema all over her skin and the speed at which God worked on her to prove that He was with me.

I have kept in contact with this family since the healing. I spoke with Melanie in May 2020, and she said her skin was still in beautiful, perfect condition, making it over three years of God stepping into her case. God left her with a lifelong testimony of His perfection in His works, and that was permanent. I give God almighty all the glory for all these testimonies. He's done it. He just placed me there so that He could put His word in my mouth and so that I could tell the world that there is really a balm in Gilead for us to believe in.

◯ October 2016 ⦿

October 2016: Supernatural Healing, Surgery Operation Cancelled — Leah, Queen's Hospital, Romford, East London

In September 2016, I enrolled to study level 7 MBA in health and social studies at Anglia Ruskin University, where I met Lara, who was also in the same course as me. However, on 29 October 2016, I went to Queen's Hospital in Romford to visit Leah, my colleague who had been in the hospital for about two weeks. I took a bottle of anointed oil with me. On my arrival at the hospital, I anointed the grounds of the hospital, starting from the gates of the hospital, and I began to pray for everyone who was sick in that hospital before entering the ward to see Leah.

When I began praying for my colleague, a word from God almighty came to me: **'You will not have any operation.'**

I could not utter a word at first because I got a rush of thoughts flooding into my head: **'Who do you think you are to give such inaccurate information?'**

Leah was admitted into the hospital for kidney problems, and the doctors had already informed Leah that she would be operated on before they would discharge her, so they were getting her ready for the surgery. However, before the fear could consume me to total numbness, I received an instruction from God to deliver the word to Leah.

Then I heard the Holy Spirit speaking to me, saying, **'You don't have to do anything. Just speak the word that I put in you.'**

As soon as it dawned on me that these words were from God to Leah and not mine to keep, I knew that they were not coming from me. I then made bold declarations, and the following words jumped out of my mouth: **'You will not have any operation. The Lord wants you to be pain free. Your healing is permanent. Father Lord, may the grace that you have upon my bishop, Oyedepo, and my pastor, Nicolas Udoh, fall upon me that there shall be testimony from this healing. This, I pray in the name of Jesus Christ. Amen.'**

I don't even know if what I was saying was making any sense, but I honestly was not calculating my speech as I spoke or didn't know if my words were coherent in the order that they dropped out of my mouth. One thing I did do and recalled for sure was that after I prayed, I committed the utterance from my mouth to God. It became clear to me that because these words were from God, they were not for me to keep to myself, but they had to be spoken to Leah, and God had sent me to deliver them for her healing. I felt a different kind of freeness within me once I emptied myself of what God had filled me with. Before I left the hospital, I gifted Leah with the bottle of anointing oil. I told her to drink it and to rub it also on her body before going to bed if she felt comfortable doing so.

The following morning, I got a text message from my colleague Leah, and it read, **'Thank you very much. The oil really worked. This is the first time I'm using it. The aches that were preventing me from sleeping all this while have left me, and last night, I did not even know when I slept.'**

On 1 November, I got another text message from Leah telling me that she had been discharged home, and no operation of any kind was made on her. On Tuesday, 15 November 2016, I received a phone call from Leah, and she began her greetings to me with thanksgiving. She thanked me in both English and Nigeria's Yoruba language; I was really flabbergasted and taken unaware because I honestly could not capture in my mind that she could still be thanking me for the prayers and God's miracle.

Ironically, I pleaded with Leah to tell me what I had done lately to warrant such gratitude because by the time of her call, I had genuinely forgotten that I had gone to pray for her; at least, the subject was not apparent in my mind until Leah started speaking. She told me that she had not only been discharged home. She added that she had also been able to return to work and had gone back to complete her studies. As if that was not enough, she also said that the doctors had dismissed all operations and that all the hospital follow-up consultants had been discharged.

This was God's miracle, and I knew it. I gave thanks to God with Leah over the phone, and then when the call ended, I later called Pastor Nicolas Udoh and told him that God was embarrassing me with so many testimonies. I confessed that I couldn't count how many testimonies I'd been blessed with daily. Pastor Nicolas Udoh advised me to begin to write them down, so I began to email my testimonies to myself as well as share some at the church.

Whenever I go out to evangelise to people about the love of Jesus Christ and His gift of salvation for them, if I discover that they are experiencing challenges or held back by disbelief of any kind, I share some of the testimonies God has blessed me with just to encourage them into believing and to boost their faith in the creative God almighty.

Leah's supernatural healing occurred in 2016. I spoke with Leah on 24 April 2020, and her healing from God is still permanent to this day. So shall it be in the mighty name of Yeshua Hamashiach. I give all the glory to God almighty, the creator of the universe.

◯ July 2016 🌐

July 2016: Exception (Soul Winning + Exemption) — Ms Christine, Dartford, Kent, England

In July 2016, I was just about to graduate from my very first Bible certificate course, but the second half of the course meant that we had to go out into the field and win souls for Christ. I remember being covered with fear. The enemy that instigated fear in my spirit was holding my past counts to account in my present work for God.

I heard from my conscious mind that if I ventured on, this would be the most humiliating adventure of my life. The critics were coming on very strongly that I would be laughed at, and nobody would listen to me because in that community where I lived at Woolwich, everyone who knew me knew me as a wayward child. Still, I got empowered by the grace of God. I suddenly spoke out to myself, saying, **'Well, that is the old me. They will need to know the new me now.'**

I was instantly transformed and charged onto the streets and announced to the world that Jesus Christ is my Lord and saviour. I went on telling this to all I met so much to the extent that I lost track of time. I and my soul-winning partner, Christine, were left behind to make our way back; there was no way for the others to contact us as we had left our bags, purses, and phones behind in the hall, as instructed by our lecturers.

I and Christine had to make our way back to the premises as fast as we could to catch up with the rest of the students, and the fastest way to get back was to use the train services. However, to use the train services, we needed to use a preloaded card to cover our travel fare. I ran to my house, which was not far from the centre where we were spreading the good news to people; I grabbed two Oyster travel cards and was unsure of how much credits they had on them.

Before we got on the train service, I said a prayer for God to guide our journey; I had no idea what would come of it, but I trusted God that we would be able to meet up with the remaining students. To my greatest surprise, as soon we began our journey, two uniformed ticket inspectors got into the train replacement bus and were inspecting the tickets of every passenger, and whoever was found without a ticket would be issued with a huge fine.

I remember seeing the wardens first and then getting Christine's attention; it felt like we had no way out should our cards be found empty. I was led to pray that they would disappear. It sounds funny now that I am narrating it to you, but then I was in a desperate state of mind for Christine should her card be found empty; I scanned mine at the entrance, and because of the panic to get back quickly, she forgot to scan hers. The only prayer that I could think of praying was a single prayer in the name of Jesus Christ that they would all disappear at once after they came in. To my amazement, I did not see these inspectors until we got off the bus train replacement service.

Now we arrived at our final destination in Kent, which is not in London, and we had been travelling from London. There was a different set of inspectors this time, standing by the barriers to restrict the movements of people who had no tickets. I remember walking straight up to the men at the gate and narrating my story to them, and to my amazement yet again, they opened the gate and let us walk through without any further questions or harassment. To this day, I thank God for His favour, which prevailed on that day.

Look out for the chapters of this book with the wonderful testimonies of God, who is the doer of every song and wonder in our lives: 'Behold, I and the children whom the LORD hath given me are for signs and wonders in Israel from the LORD of hosts, which dwelleth in Mount Zion' **(Isaiah 8:18)**. 'Our hope is not in the rainbow but in the one who put the colours in the rainbow.'

Chapter VII

 NEW BEGINNINGS

Beginnings

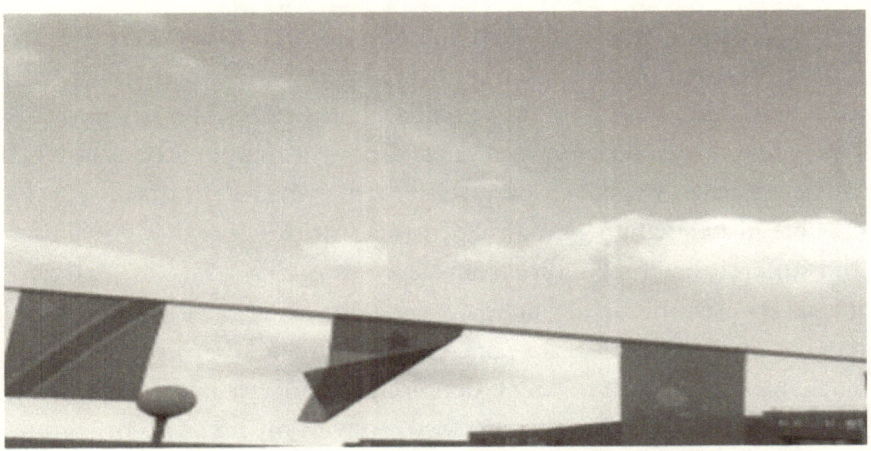

From the time we run into the end of the road, where the enemy has pursued us – this is the beginning of the road where God starts with us for a new beginning. A true statement from the late Benson Idahosa, the archbishop of Church of God Mission International, in one of his videos is the following: 'Every time you're seriously sick, the devil leaves a mark behind, and every time you're seriously injured, there is a scar left behind. But when God turns your scar into a star, that's when you start jumping and praising.'

Real-life stories are really cheesy to read, right? The reason this is so, among many other reasons, could be that when you tell your story, people cannot believe how cruel people can be to one another and how much a person goes through in life, hopping over different battles in life, and can remain standing. I figured out that it does not matter if people believe my story or not when I tell it to them. The most important thing is that I have shared my experience with them and that a part of my life that would aid in their journey in life has been made freely available to them as a means of them coming in contact and getting in touch with the testimonies that have formed my books. However, in the midst of all the life challenges I have been through, my hope still remains in the promises of God almighty; whether I find myself in the deep or shallow end of the waters, I have stretched myself to lean unto the Most High for His strength.

In my journey of going through one obstacle to another, I have heard some people tell me that I am an overcomer, while others have called me a hero; most have said I am a walking miracle, but I know now that I have no powers to keep myself alive. I always give glory back to God. However, when I was at a period in my life when I felt that I was not capable of believing in anything in this world, I was living in limbo and suffered much brutality from depression. The grace of God kept me sane even when I did not give reverence to Him. I suffered more low moods for a long period once upon a time. Then I found myself stuck in a tunnel without any vision or light until one faithful day when I looked back on my life to move forward with my life, with or without soundness in my health, and this was when I took myself out from the victim's box to the victorious box.

Think yourself victorious and not a victim even when being victimised. I began to see myself as victorious even when I was still in the midst of the hellish circumstances all around me, circumstances that battled with my health and wealth to see that I never got off the ground. Still, my God gave me a hand up and lifted me off the ground, and I no longer see myself as a loser but a winner in spite of what battle the enemy throws my way.

It is not easy to overcome a difficult period of pain in life because when a lot of painful emotions pass through the human body, they leave feelings of pain, anger, and sorrow; sometimes it is better to be dead than to be alive so that all the negative emotions would be frozen up. I know this feeling because I too have felt it several times in the past. These feelings were more apparent in my life when I had no idea of the reason for my creation and why the enemy was fighting me. So in a sense, I had no idea of who I really was as I was not identifying with the creative God of heaven and earth.

In the Beginning

When I began to hear from God more frequently than usual at the beginning of the year 2020, I became more conscious of my sinful behaviour. The more conscious I became of sinful patterns in my life, the more I heard from God to separate myself from the parcels and persons that looked good but were bad for my personal and spiritual development.

Chapter 1 in this book makes mention of how God found the world first before He created the whole wide world in the beginning; drawing from this, everything has a beginning, middle, and end, just like each day has a start, which gives us a new opportunity to start the day with fresh grace for the race ahead. The beginning of a journey determines the end of that journey; this is why it is important to map out the journey ahead before venturing out to avoid getting lost while on the journey. Although preparation does not take away disappointment or surprises, it, puts a person one step ahead of any opponent. However, with the lack of planning in the beginning, one is doomed to fail. Going back to God's creation, in the beginning, God created; when He created, He said, 'Let there be light,' and today no manner of evil can shut down the light of God.

At the start of each new year, we also have a beginning, where we find that a lot of people make new year vows of what changes they want to see happen in their lives. However, sometimes, because of certain distractions in life, the majority of people with good will and intentions are not always able to maintain these vows and promises because of distractions, which come in different forms and shapes. This can, in essence, make it seem as if not everything is under our control.

In the beginning, destinies are created. So it is better to have your destiny constructed at the beginning of the year in the presence of the Lord to enable the Holy Spirit to orchestrate your life. This is so that you can step into your victorious place in life that has been assigned for you from the beginning of your creation.

For example, when you commit your destiny in God's hands at the start of the year, you are entrusting God to secure your destiny for you with the knowing that He will not mismanage it. This way, you are partnering with God with a sense of responsibility in knowing that while God is doing His part, you have to do your part also. For this reason, it is important to come into the presence of the Lord at the beginning of the new year, also so that you and the Holy Spirit can both have that initial agreement of that which is in God's covenant. See how you relate with God – not as a religion but as a spiritual activity.

In this sense, you are committing God's hands to take your hand, and you begin this with your words and actions: **'Lord, I trust you with this plan of mine because it is from you, so you are in it. I trust that you will deliver and see me through to the end of it and take me to my place of destiny without mishandling it because it is your desire that I prosper.'**

234

As a believer, you will be taking conscious steps and be deliberate about those decisions that you have committed in God's hands. Know that entering a relationship with God is partnering with Him. Now you have the mentality that when you're coming into the new year partnering with God, you already have and feel that sense of responsibility that while God is doing His part, ensuring that your life will be fulfilled with His plan for you, you are committed to doing your bit to see that your actions are in line with the plan God has for you so that you can remain in the process for your consistent progress.

That's why it is very important in the beginning of the year to come under His presence – so you can both have that initial agreement so that when you start backsliding or falling back on your part, you have that support and lift in His word and from His revelations to you. The revelations are what are revealed to you by the Holy Spirit the moment you come into His presence in praise and prayer.

Revelations are paradise's equivalent of conversations as they are the conversations you have directly with God, which empower you to acquire your possessions as you've had them revealed to you, having followed the instructions that were given to you following the revelation. This is not by your might; you are only empowered by the strength of God almighty, and when you humble yourself to receive what the Spirit of God is giving to you, it is then that God breathes His wisdom into your lungs and gives you new ideas and inspiration to go ahead with your goals in life.

As established in the beginning of this section, what happens in the beginning of an adventure determines how the end of that adventure is going to turn out. Even in cooking, if the food is overly salted at the start of cooking, no matter how much water you pour into the pot, the food would not taste as delicious as you intended it to be but will rather lose its taste because it's been watered down. This is why it is ideal to plan your recipe before you begin cooking – so you can gauge what measurements of food ingredients you will need to add. In the same vein, when we are stepping into the new year, let's not take it for granted and narrow the celebration as a 'fireworks' type of event. Yes, you can have fireworks if you want it this way, but this can be so any time of the year, so why not light up the most important fire in your life, which is the one in your soul, and have your life enlightened for the rest of the year by inviting the Holy Spirit to dwell in it?

I came to realise this at the early stage of my walk with God, when I had some understanding of what it means to give my life to God. My celebration of entering into the new year changed because yes, the fireworks go up with a bang, but when the light goes out (talking about my own experience), my mood goes down. However, this was not so when God's light lit up my life because no man can shut down the light of God in me, just like a candle cannot be hidden under the mattress when lit; in this case, it would be seen as a fire hazard as the light must surely find a way to express its spark. So when found in a person, the light of God just keeps on firing up in them, up and up, going from glory to glory until the glorious day of Jesus's return.

Beginning to End

To see the end of a beginning, you must adapt the attitude to apply consistency no matter the challenge. Be persistent in your growth no matter the odds within the challenge. Insist that you must prevail in the midst of the challenge no matter the external forces forcing you to remain in the same circle of the challenge. Most importantly, be determined to show the challenge that God almighty is way bigger than it seems to pose over you. Remember that Jesus is the only Lord over your life. Also, don't forget to make the most of your time within the challenging circumstances. Although they may prevent you from climbing up the steps, look out for smaller stairs that you can climb, which will eventually take you to higher heights that will lead you towards where you want to get to.

Take advantage of the challenging circumstances and develop yourself from the actual challenge so that when you

leave the challenging circumstances behind, the challenge has not left you behind life events, this sway away from the challenge leaving the challenge to become a challenge onto itself.

'If the challenge will not let you go until it dies, then don't let the challenge go until you make sure it's dead so you can live with God-given peace.'

— Merisha Meisha

◯ Last Chapter ◉

During the creating process of this book, I encountered attacks on my health caused by the enemy to steal my joy and wealth. I had to restructure my life as quickly as God was enabling me to so that I would be able to complete this book in time. My mentality had to change with the way I ran my affairs, both with myself and with the people around me. I told everyone that I was working full time because I did devote my time to my writing alongside other duties in my life while developing my business as well as my creative works, some of which are seen in this book. Also, I did apply different structures to my schedule, which allowed me the flexibility to have healthy distractions so that my mind was not constantly on work. As well, determining my typing speed has given me the discipline to manage my time better.

Separately, I took time away from my writing to invite different interesting activities into my life, and I found this useful, having achieved other things while writing. However, the most challenging aspect about working on my writing project with dyslexia is that I am aware that my mind is incredibly creative, so I have to constantly find channels to box up new inspirations that pop into my thoughts so that they do not become a means of distraction. This way, I am able to work and not be distracted, and I am able to remain on the same project and not dive into another without finishing the project at hand; this method has been a key factor/point of focus throughout this book-writing process.

Another factor of this book-writing project that I would have found very sensitive to cross had I not healed from the pain is the suicide of my late brother as it was ten years ago in July. For ten solid years, I really struggled with his death, and so I boxed up a part of me regarding this matter and was unable to talk about the loss because of the stigma of suicide, highly seen as a taboo subject in most cultures around the world.

Still, *My Mental Health Matter*, this book, has given me the opportunity to express to my audience the emotions I felt through poetry on a subject that was still on my mind; I could not find a space to talk about it until I found a safe space through my writing to begin to deal with the pain. Then how long it took me to heal was an apparent subject on my mind, along with how my faith in God carried me through the healing process even when I was still broken and contemplated taking my own life. This, coupled with physical health complications, is a miracle because among everything, I tried to speed up the healing process. It was only by God's mercy and grace that I became completely free from the trauma of guilt and torment of losing someone as close to me as my brother, not because he was my brother alone but because we were close.

◉ Opening the Day with God ◉

I had to be selfish with my timing so that I could catch up with my workload for the day, read, and do sports and relaxation, all in the daytime. Bearing this in mind, if I started my day by looking at my phone, I would never accomplish what I set out to gain, so I made sure that I did not sleep with my phone beside me, and at most, I removed it from the room I slept in at night. I had to set aside time for everything, as if I was going to work outdoors, so that my walking time did not affect my working time.

As soon as I open my eyes in the morning, I open my mouth and begin to thank God for brining me into the land of the living and for keeping me alive all throughout the night, right up to the new day. I then reach for the window and begin to thank God for the dawning of the morning. This gratitude graduates to the bathroom, where I then sing a thanksgiving song as a mark of entering the day with God from my heart into my house.

When you sing to the creator of the universe first thing in the morning, you are telling the devil that none of his tricks will pull you down as well as renewing your joy. You are also putting on the armour of God because you are building up your faith from the songs you're singing by telling God you know He remains the mightiest of the mighty. The enemy, who may be eavesdropping, will hear your song; their arrows will be extinguished because you know who you are, and the God whom you serve is heartily engaged in your affairs.

Even if we are in our homes, we still have to enter the new day with the fresh attitude of entering the presence of God because we have new applications to God daily, just as His daily benefits to us are new every day. So to present this application, we would need to apply an appreciation of who He is.

◯ Revealed ◉

Revelations kept me going in the year 2020. No matter where I turned, God was just there, waiting for me with a word from heaven. Among some of the words I received from the divine heavens are shown below, and they kept me typing one more chapter during times I felt like giving up. ***There are so many of them, but a few are shown below.***

- 'Can two walk together, except they be agreed?' **(Amos 3:3)**
- 'The Spirit of God had made me, and [the] breath of the Almighty hath given me life.' **(Genesis 2:7)**
- 'By your strips, I am healed.' **(Isaiah 53:5)**
- 'I and my children and my husband are for signs and wonders.' **(Isaiah 8:18)**
- 'I am she who lives alive. Have you heard?' **(John 11:25)**

- 'Whatever He tells you to do, do it.' **(John 2:5)**
- 'I must do the works of my Father in the day time.' **(John 9:4)**
- 'Blessed is she who has believed that the Lord would fulfill His promises to her, for there shall be a performance.' **(Luke 1:45)**
- 'The light of the body is the eye; if therefore thine eye be single, thy whole body shall be full of light.' **(Matthew 6:22)**
- 'Stay with me. I am with you always so don't be afraid to do whatever I ask you to do.' **(Matthew 28:20)**
- 'There are so many afflictions on the righteous but the Lord delivers him out of them all.' **(Psalms 34:19)**
- 'But the path of the just is as the shining light that shineth more and more unto the perfect day.' **(Proverbs 4:18)**

◐ Dedicated Discipline ◉

Discipline is a self-applied element that complements a person's attempt to accomplish their mission. No matter the dedication in practice, if the theory learned is not in action, then the discipline is not complete. My determination to complete this book alone wasn't enough to keep me focused on my writing because there were times when other life factors came flooding in as important, but I had to ask for help in these areas. Sometimes I even cried out for help, and it took the inspiration of the Holy Ghost to help me get through such moments. Nevertheless, inasmuch as the Holy Spirit is my friend, teacher, and guide, it down to me to use my pen to see that the works went into print. **While planning, take steps – 'tick by tock', like the clock. This way, you talk and do.**

God has already gone ahead to see that your movement is fast-tracked, but you have to take the first step. Being dedicated in our duties does not mean jumping into the deep end straight away. Setting ourselves up for reasonable, achievable tasks so that we don't set ourselves up to fail is an ideal practice for success. Take steps. The staircase is long, but your foot is all you need to take the first step, and God will lift you up. Rather than looking for the lift before you move, use the stairs; what if the lift is broken and you then have to go back to the stairs and climb up with your God-given legs?

The trees we see today make a forest tomorrow because the arborist first had the idea to plant. Then he got the seeds and took further steps to dig into the ground before pouring the seeds into the soil. He did not stop there; he watered the ground over the seeds and then built a net around the area of the plantation so that the birds of the air or other creatures of the earth would not dig out the seeds. This planter did not stop nurturing these seeds until they formed trees that grew branches, which became a forest. So don't be stuck in your thoughts because they are giants waiting to come out, even if they may look like ants at the moment. However, to help those thoughts become giants, you need to take gentle steps; otherwise, they will remain trapped in the mind, like ants waiting to escape from a hole under the ground.

Refusing to take steps to move is what causes one to feel small, which warrants thoughts of feeling small to grip the person in frustration. So taking these gentle steps to meet our goals is very important for us to move with the idea when it comes, but first, present it to God for the leading of the Holy Ghost. When taking steps, set yourself up with achievable, reasonable tasks so as not to fail. Even if the idea is a big one, take an aspect of it that is small and begin with that so that it will grow with you while you're still in your set goal.

Imagine that you can't jump from the ground to reach the top of a tree at once. There is a procedure to climb up it. Unless you have been trained to have such a skill for years, an attempt of this can lead to an accident that will make you end up with some fractures/injuries. This is a metaphorical example of the consequence of trying to run before walking but is not limited to when God grants an individual speed. When God grants speed, He enables and equips the individual to take off at once.

◯ Timing ◉

In terms of disciplining my timing, I made myself account for every single second per minute per hour. I then made a commitment and said to God almighty that I would make it my duty to spend my time cautiously, keeping each new day that He added to my life. This way, I knew that even if I had been given the freedom to use my time, I still had to account to God how I had used it because my time is God's time; even though my freedom is mine, my time remains His.

I became adamant that there would not be any wasted minute, and no single hour would be idle. This is a bit like being in a working environment, where you have the lunch hour and tea breaks, all paid for. In such a setting, every single second is recorded, including and especially break times; they are clocked in and clocked out on the system so that the payment is accurate and the staff members are not self-ruled.

Bearing this in mind, I developed a mentality that made me fully acknowledge God as both my 'boss man' and *oga* to report to, and I had to be conscious of the fact that I was constantly making progress with my engagements towards the completion of my book project. This way, I felt that I was fulfilling my purpose, and what's more, I have a supreme, supernatural, divine living God who cares that I am productive and progressive while processing the information I am receiving through the inspiration of the Holy Spirit.

My time is still God's time; this is why He accounts for it in the end of my days. So I took the responsibility to put in a structure that allows me to take practical measures for maintaining this habit so that I can master a completely pressure-free way of mixing my working, eating, exercising, and play time as well as creating room for certain people who are important in my life and I in theirs. Putting myself in a routine puts me at ease with my work daily. Yes, some days do not go according to plan, and I have to reschedule, but that is part of the beauty of life. We don't always know what will be thrown at us, but preparing ahead makes life easier to handle unexpected events in life.

It is easier to readjust. Although it is almost impossible to prepare for everything because all is not revealed to us at once, it is OK to accept this aspect of life because it is in the nature of God, to whom secrets belong. Having said that, being prepared mentally makes it easier to zoom forward with life's surprising moments.

Sometimes something uncontrollable will come from the outside that would force a drastic shift to occur. Dynamics like these force us to move from a position unannounced, but they never leave us completely out of control because the decision is still down to us, and it is the choices that we make that make the difference of what we will encounter next in our journey of life. Notice how I did not say 'how things turn out' because in this life, there are so many forces taking charge over us, but an intensive focus on what we are working towards is what transports us to see that things happen the way we visualise them to happen. Otherwise, time would be wasted as we work without a focus on the goal.

Putting zero tolerance on saying yes to random social invitations and visitations during working hours is a key time management strategy. Imagine the things you are not allowed to do when you are employed by an organisation; don't do them when you are self-employed or working directly for God in your ministry. This is not to suggest that you cannot leave the room for spontaneous events, but such events needs to be calculated and fit in with your work so that your efficiency remains articulated.

Basically saying a simple 'No, thank you' is very powerful. So saying 'No, thanks' to a random invitation is within my power to do. This also goes for an official last-minute invitation from the board; that means having to drop everything that I am working on, which has a set date to submit. I too can exercise my rights and say, **'No, thank you. I am working on a very important project that is taking up my time and very pressing for me to complete. Mind if we reschedule, please?'** Most likely, they will beg you to accept or reschedule if you are really needed in that meeting. So don't feel pressured to accept every invitation that may remove you from producing your own product.

On the contrary, if an unexpected invitation comes in that will add fruitfulness to what you are working towards, then appropriate discretion is needed to apply the right application so as to avoid any distractions that will steal time unnecessarily. Additionally, on time discipline (those steps that we take towards achieving the things that we set out to do so that we are not stagnant), we have to set for ourselves reasonable, achievable tasks that permit us to move gradually with time to accomplish our mission.

◎ Inspiration ◉

My inspiration comes from the divine heavens above. When I commit my creative works to the Holy Spirit, I hear the Holy Spirit telling me what to write. Even when I don't know what it means, I jot it down. Then later, the Holy Spirit brings the translation to me in pictures or in other words. To my greatest amazement, when I look up the meaning, it fits exactly what I am conveying in theory.

◎ Language ◉

In the year 2020, I was going to take my English course again, and I was concerned about the studious aspect of it.

I heard the Holy Ghost tell me, 'Sit down. I am going to teach you.'

I chuckled when I heard this, not because it was unbelievable but because of the dimension in which I received this message. I moved quickly in the direction of something, which, for most people, would be an act of madness. That was what made me laugh – because I believed it straight away, even if I could hear a small voice from my spirit saying, 'How?' I ran to the WHSmith bookstore and bought myself a notepad that came with a pen that read on its front cover 'Write Away'.

I was taught by the Holy Ghost some fundamental words that I needed to write down. Even before I thought deeply about a word I had never heard before, it was deposited into my heart to fit into the exact sentence that I wanted to write in that section of my writing, to the point of amazement because when I searched the word up on Google, it was an actual word that was coherent with my paragraph.

I kept hearing the most incredible words that I never thought I would ever come in contact with in my life by searching through the dictionary because I would not even know what it meant, let alone search it online.

I remember telling Sister Faith, 'The Holy Spirit is talking to me again.'

She said, 'Write it down.'

◯ Eating ◉

Food is only as important as you make it. Just like people, it is the attention you give it that makes it attractive to you. I spent less time thinking of what to eat and more time in thoughts of when to write because what to write always formed plenty of thoughts in my head, but food, most times, got in the way and stole some of my writing time.

My discipline with food did not happen overnight, just like how my discipline from social media did not happen overnight. This habit to fast as a lifestyle so that I would not be led by food ate me up. Rather, eating food when I decided to came gradually. I am still working on it, just as I am still working on everything else in my life. Life is a work in progress, and the day we stop working on ourselves is the day our footprints are written off the sands.

I forced myself to fast on the days when food almost swallowed me up just to prove that food was made for me to eat, not for me to be eaten. In so doing, I could last in fasting as long as I desired, stretching myself further sometimes just to have that grip over food. Minding my eating helped me avoid eating in random places or getting lost over food in certain times. It also encouraged me to reflect on how I ate and what

I ate so that I could select good food for consumption instead of being consumed by food.

Sports

At the beginning of the year 2020, I went to my local leisure centre to enquire about a swimming membership. My aim was to use swimming as one of my fitness exercises, but because of COVID-19, the swimming pool remained closed for the rest of the year, so I began to take my walking exercise more seriously. Walking daily became part of my routine, and I used part of my walking time and turned it into a prayer to praise God. *Walking for six miles two and a half hours a day became a normal routine for me.*

Health

The more I progressed with my writing, the more the enemy (the devil and his agents) became vicious and unhappy to see me progress in spite of my challenges. The enemy is never happy to see us prosper in good health, and definitely when we are happy, the enemy is very angry to see us getting on with our God-given project, especially the one that is aligned with our destiny and that God has blessed us with in our hands.

Remember that God comes to give life more abundantly, but the enemy comes to steal and to destroy. God has access to us to bless us; in the same way, the enemy finds ways to sneak in and hurt us. So when we hear the word 'the enemy', let us not freak out as if it's some monster that only resides six feet under the ground. Nope. There are wicked household persons and evil principalities crafting our destinies. They are known as the compound witches and wizards within our circle who come with the faces of friends and family to help Satan complete his mission. Still, this is not to suggest that every friend and family member is such.

The biggest lie that satanic agents want people to believe, especially in European countries, is that there are no witches so that they can keep operating on their victims underground and keep them hostage, with no room for escape. If you don't believe the above statement, ask J. K. Rowling. Also, have you ever wondered why the scriptures talk about sorcerers and witches if they do not exist? If this were false, then this indicates that the whole scripture is based on false information.

The trick of the enemy is to base unseen battles and demonic attacks on mental health disorderliness so that authentic intervention is void. This way, help is denied, and torment is extended because the battles are almost invisible to onlookers, yet the after-effects are publically noticed by natural eyes.

◯ Sex and the Sin Thing ◉

We are bought for a price. This means that our bodies are not ours but the Lord's. Therefore, we must summit our body temples to their creator for the reasons He designed them for and have them kept sacred for us until we are married. It is not until we are married that we are legitimately permitted to intimately explore our sexual desires with our spouse. Anything we do sexually with our bodies outside marriage defiles our bodies and makes us drop down spiritual heights.

Until we understand this, it will be hard to walk in obedience of this law, and sexual sin would be almost impossible for us to overcome because it will pose as a god before our eyes; until understanding in this area comes alive, one will not see the light in this truth. Therefore, for as long as the light is off in this area of our lives, the enemy will keep on sneaking in through the sin gap left open here.

When I was growing up, I distanced myself from boys because I felt intimidated by them, but later on in my teenage years, I thought this timid, so I began to make friends with boys but kept them on the other side of the bridge and kept anything sexual away from our relationship. On the contrary, when forming sexual relationships with the opposite sex, as I am female, I don't know how to be in a casual relationship, and from the get-go, there has always seemed to be a serious commitment to settle down for life in marital bliss.

In 2020, God took me through thorough discipline on sexual habits and about the severity of sexual immorality. In the same year, He taught me, through the help of the Holy Spirit, about practicing daily cleansing in the region of my vagina. Moreover, to perfect His work in this area of my life, Jesus Christ, the king of all kings, used this channel of sanitising to purify me internally and externally. This sanctification terminated my bad on-and-off masturbation habit that had lived with me all of my life, to end with no trace or desire of reoccurrence until eternity.

Whatever God does, He perfects it. Masturbation had been an issue for me for as far back as I could remember, to the extent where I preferred masturbating over gaining sexual pleasure from a male companion. I tried to stop because I used to spend hours trying to please myself sexually. Pleasing myself and imagining my partner as if it were him in action was a normal, sweet thing for me, but this is the plan of the devil to hold down the destinies of people. ***Know or believe it or not, but best believe that masturbation is a time bomb set for the destruction of glorious destinies.***

I remember trying what I knew as my best to quit masturbating in 2017. When the temptation came back in 2018, I overcame it and ran to share the testimony of how I had been able to stop masturbating after I brought this issue to God during seven days of fasting and praying. Yes, I had stopped masturbating because I used the 'I must stop it' willpower of my mind to maintain this stand, but my body always sent a different message to my brain, hence causing sexual arousal to be the order of the day, especially when I was alone. The feelings came on very strong; I use to contemplate whether it would be better to have an orgasm to release any sexual tension that was building up in my body.

Friends, the fight to stop masturbating is real and is on for thousands of believers all round the world. It got to me to the extent where I had to wrestle with my mind to keep my focus, but the grace of God sustained me and kept me from falling for feelings of the flesh, masturbating my day away, sliding into the hole of temptation by the trick master, who is the devil.

The grapple to be free completely from the temptation of masturbating kept reoccurring in the fashion described above until May 2020, when I experienced an episode of insomnia. It felt as if every single muscle in my body had locked up, and the only way I could unlock it and be tension free was to masturbate. This was not the only issue; the next beautiful thing that happened in not-so-good timing (when without spouse) was that I felt incredibly horny without anything triggering sexual excitement.

Not knowing what to do with my sexual feelings, I ran to Uncle Google to search my way out of masturbating. I carefully keyed in search things like 'Is masturbating a sin?' It was almost as if I actually wanted a reason to masturbate yet be reassured that God would not be upset with me for touching my body indecently. However, the more I ventured on in my search, the more often I came across this scripture:

'No temptation has overtaken you except what is common to mankind. And God is faithful; He will not let you be tempted beyond what you can bear. But when you are tempted, He will also provide a way out so that you can endure it.' (1 Corinthians 10:13, New International Bible)

Surely, God would not give me a temptation that I could not handle. I had been using the above scripture previously but not consistently to run away from the temptation of playing with myself. but longer nights shifted into days, and I found myself still awake, tempted to touch myself. I tried to get into my daily activity and keep myself on top of things as much as I could, but given the mixture of the lack of sleep with everything else and tension in my muscles, I became weak.

I soon could not take the struggle of fighting off my libido any longer, so I discovered that taking myself to bed and resting with my eyes closed was a good distraction for some minutes until the sexual desires shifted away from my body. This was occurring more than I could handle because I was losing time just waiting for my body not to be aroused before I could resume my activities. This method affected my timing and schedule, so I decided to take my sexual matter to my space in the therapy room so that it could be addressed. To be honest, I was losing work time trying to sleep the feelings away, but the feelings did not slide away, so I had to think of something else that would help me stop masturbating.

Uncontrollably, after I felt so much pressure on my body from not sleeping after a few nights, I became desperate to get a solution for my sleep, having tried a few other things that could have helped but did not instantly help. I wanted a quick stimulus response to react in my body and send me to sleep at once for a few hours with no interruptions. This desperation took me back to the masturbation that I had left years ago but had not completely left me; hence, it would not have been an option for me to consider.

My body was demanding something that it was receiving, but at the same time, my mind was rejecting it so that my body could not receive the pleasure that it demanded from me. Hence, I was masturbating but not climaxing. I noticed that I was forcing myself to masturbate so I could feel sleepy after climaxing but not enjoying it. I was getting annoyed that my search for sleep had resulted to masturbating, and it still was not working, especially because I thought this was a closed chapter in my life.

Something scary happened to me one day while I was masturbating. I heard a voice say, 'I will destroy you.' It was so scary; I took caution at once, but it did not stop there. Just after a few days, I began to try sleeping again through masturbation with the hope that I would become dizzy after and then fall asleep. Can you imagine that, hearing that you would be destroyed for masturbating? That still did not make me stop immediately, knowing that there was a very strong evil force behind masturbating. I went back to God to beg for forgiveness. I also began to remind God that He is capable of providing all my needs, including my sexual needs.

Although masturbating for me this time around was not down to sexual frustration, I reminded God to take care of my sexual needs anyway because I did not want to pray to stop feeling sexual; I wanted God to deliver me from masturbation once and for all. I knew that God was more than capable of going beyond all my expectations, but my faith needed to grow in this area so that God could do it even if I didn't know how He would do it. ***God is more than able to provide all my needs, including my sexual needs. How He does it is miraculous and marvellous in our eyes.***

While I was building my faith to trust God with my sleep and sex life, I was still in sin. On 19 May 2020 – in the afternoon, to be precise – I began masturbating again; floods of thoughts rushed into my brain. I really needed help and did not know where to start when I could have just called on the Holy Ghost to get me out; I began to think of a way out from this sinking ship. I was in the middle of the act when I felt so remorseful and ashamed of myself and began to think of how I had let myself down and disobeyed God. Right in the middle of my thoughts, a deep sense of regret came upon me. While I was lost in myself, in the middle of my mess, I got a raw revelation from God.

'What has a child got to do with masturbating?' was what I heard.

I paused and thought, 'What?'

The next line went like this: 'This has held you back. It's a plague.'

Hearing this took me a few waves back into my childhood. I remembered I had been masturbating as a child; it did not make sense, and I still can't think of any special way of telling how that part of me had ever begun. My answer and total deliverance came on this day, and God sealed this deliverance following an instruction and a love letter. I got another opportunity to rededicate my life to God.

I was instructed to be consistent in maintaining personal cleansing to allow the Holy Ghost to purify me. Since Jesus Christ took me through this sanctification, I had been shown how to maintain my virginity. I felt the sanitising of the Holy Spirit from the inside out, and this made me feel lighter and happy without any concerns of any kind of uncontrollable sexual desires that could lead to any thoughts of masturbating or feelings of indulging in sexual immorality of any kind with another.

The devil always wants to defile the finished work of God by all means, and he will use any living or non-living thing to get his way; that's how stubborn he is. After I got my release from this ordeal, males came out from all kinds of woodwork to show that they wanted to be sexually active regardless of the coronavirus as if not having sex was my challenge. Some even acted as if they wanted to do me a favour until they found about the God who keeps me all round.

I've been asked numerous times to reveal my secret, and my answer will never change: 'It is God.' The mystery remains hard for some people to understand because they are yet to encounter light in this area. They still look on as if I would pull something out from my bag and say, 'This is it,' but the truth is that it is not that my body is wooden; it is that I handed it over to God, and He helps sustain me physically, mentally, and sexually. How I got out of this atrocity can only be because of God. If you have received this type of miracle, you too can resonate with the testimony of God's intervention because masturbating can leave the individual seriously addicted and secluded.

On 5 June 2020, at 6:00 a.m., my love letter from God arrived, delivered and personally addressed to me, as I read Isaiah 54 ('My most precious love, Merisha . . .'). This scripture kept reminding me of God's promises for me as well as strengthened me to know the God who is on my side and who I am. I truly am kept safe and sound knowing this without any obscurity in this department of my life.

Is it true that some believers suffer from masturbation but still, if they had to disclose this secret habit and so forth, continue to suffer behind closed doors rather than confide in the trustworthy supernatural/spiritual head (Jesus) so that they can be healed? *If you have not yet received your deliverance from masturbating and you desire to be free from this bondage. I pray that God will deliver you from it today in the mighty name of Jesus Christ. In addition, God will bless you with a good life partner and make your marriage productive and fruitful for His glory. If you are already married, in your marriage, your sexual desires shall be satisfied.*

Some may argue that 'it is their body' and they can do what they like. Supporting this statement, I have heard people saying that before they became Christian, first, they were born with a gender type, and as Tasha J. puts it, people should not be bound to a religion, and so they can choose their sexual orientation and live their lives the way they decide. My reply to Tasha's statement will remain that before you were born, He who created you knew what you would become, and He formed you for a reason. See what He said to Jeremiah below. Remember what He says to one, He is still saying to all.

Dr Paul Eneche of Dunamis Church addressed this subject of us claiming the self as ours in his Seeds of Destiny daily devotional (14 July 2021 edition), **_'Not Taken By Surprise'._** Dr Paul Eneche reminds us in his own words, 'Your arrival on the earth did not take God by surprise.' He goes further: 'The scripture makes it clear that Our God does not act randomly. He is a God who acts deliberately', as seen in **Jeremiah 1:5: 'Before I formed thee in the belly, I knew thee; and before thou camest forth out of the womb, I sanctified thee, and I ordained thee a prophet unto the nations.'**

Going back to Tasha's statement at the top, living how we like does not sound like a guarantee to a profound life. As such, no good and responsible parent would want their children to live carelessly, hence why there are set rules in every home that wants to see the success of their family. We are not called into a religion but to journey with Christ in a relationship and live like Christ. Hence, believers are called Christians because their lifestyle should reflect a Christlike way of living, so what is not found in Christ should not be traced in believers of Christ. Emphasising on this point, let's hear what Dominion, a Christian brother, said in his testimony of how he got freed from masturbating.

In November 2019, I heard a testimony from Dominion. W. Dominion's testimony made my eyebrows rise up, almost above my forehead, because of the explicit, graphic image captured as he spoke. I began to imagine that if Jesus Christ had never been heard of masturbating, then how was it found in us? If you cannot imagine this in Jesus Christ, know that it is not for you already.

Dominion shared that he was delivered from masturbation after he saw a naked madman on the street stroking his dick up and down in a public and busy road. People became ecstatic by the sight of this, and this made various people display all manner of behaviours in their expression of shock. Dominion's reaction was an impetuous one as he explained that seeing the actions of the madman made his stomach turn, and as a reaction, he began to vomit instantly and recklessly. He described that in that moment, a voice spoke into his spirit, saying, **'Look at that madman. He is doing the same thing you enjoy doing.'**

So for a split second, Dominion thought himself mad to be masturbating and could not comprehend that a madman would be compared to himself. What seemed to be an exaggeration from his reaction by onlookers was a violent purging of his system from the inside out, from deep in his organs. He did not mind that people were drawing their own conclusions from his public display, and although he may have still come across as a slick guy in his public ways of life, his private lifestyle was far from it as what he did sneakily in the dark had been exposed to him as a shameful part of himself. He decided then and there that he never wanted to be associated with such shame, so he walked in partnership with the Holy Spirit to deliver him once and for all.

On reflection, Dominion's testimony made me put myself in the boat not full of mad women but with Jesus Christ, my king, living to His royal standards so I too could not be categorised as those who masturbate for any reason. I say 'any reason' because I was in denial that masturbation would help me sleep (**bear in mind that it did not for me**). I came across, during my search on this topic, information that some of the benefits include better sleep and a few others that you can actually get from improving your relationships with yourself, others, and your partner. Other areas – such as looking after your body and mind by eating better, exercising more, and connecting with your spirit – can also fulfil and improve areas in your life without any negative side effects.

For example, you can have a healthier sex life with your spouse if you both are open to discussing your sex life together as a couple to explore what is more enjoyable and then have it as you like it. If communicating this aspect of your life is an issue, you can both agree to see a sex therapist together, but be mindful of what therapist you see. I say this because if they do not practice this same Christian faith as you do, you may both be misled and end up having a wider gap in your sex life, which you should avoid at all costs. So research what the practices of the therapist are first before engaging in and investing your time and mind into their services.

You can have lots of pleasurable moments with your partner throughout the day, and this will aid your reduction of stress, release tension, and make you feel more relaxed. Adequately, you will have better sex the next time you are sexually intimate with each other because during the course of the day, you would have found out what makes either of you tick on what side by the way you tease and tickle each other.

You can introduce playful massages with each other from time to time, not just before penetrating. Building up your sexual life from the 'zero' to the 'hero' level involves both parties' engagement. Again, massaging each other regularly will make your bodies relax a bit more and boost up your mood; you both will feel loved/valued by and appreciate each other more. You will understand your sexual needs and desires better. Built-up body tension and cramps will be eased off.

After trying all that and some other sexual skills and experiences to spice up your sex life, you'll find that after all those practices, what you'll end up getting is sex made easy and enjoyable. Because you are involved romantically, you don't need to do solo masturbation that would leave behind bad side effects with traceable negative comebacks.

As already written, you can tap into the benefits in other ways and be enhanced by them, but some of the side effects are costly and could leave a person out of money in their pocket. For example, masturbating can lead to an excessive masturbating addiction, which can lead to pornography addiction; addiction steals time away from the person, and anything that steals one's time is a life thief. A lot of virtues are lost through masturbation, and the loss of virtue is equal to losing one's destined position as an individual's virtue, when secured, is the pathway that takes them to their enthronement in life.

When a person is addicted to masturbating, they are likely to become antisocial and very sensitive to sexual jokes around their partners. Being active in masturbating can also deny an individual the potential of matching with and meeting their lifelong partner because they have detached themselves from the opposite sex. This kind of sexual addiction can also make an individual isolate themselves from everyone else. There's a thin line between a person being preserved and a person being isolated; if not judged correctly, isolation for a certain period is a mental health illness.

Some people who replace real-life partners with masturbating sometimes suffer from low self-esteem, and often they themselves feel as if others think them weird because they have never been seen in a relationship. Masturbation can make a person feel a sense of wrongdoing. In other words, they feel dirty and a sense of self-pity and sometimes guilt afterwards.

If you think not, why is masturbation done in secret and not openly declared as a thing to be proud of? You have heard people talk about how sexy and sexually active their partner is, but rarely do you hear a person boasting that they are playing with themselves in the dark. For example, you can see a couple kissing in public happily because this is natural. On the other hand, if you see a person molesting themselves in public, it will be seen as madness, so why do so in hiding when God sees all, both hidden and in the open?

Masturbating while in a marital relationship can make the other person feel inadequate in satisfying their partner sexually. For some, trust can easily be lost if the other is addicted to masturbating, while for others, it can unfortunately drive them into cheating on their spouse if they feel that they have been denied their sexual due from their husband or wife.

There are critics in every subject, and some critics may criticise how it is that this side effect suggests that it is degrading to masturbate. The following synonyms from Collins Online include a few un-dignifying names for masturbating:

- **Self-abuse**
- **Wanking (taboo slang)**
- **Beating the meat**

Let us weigh the benefits of masturbating to the side effects. The negative side effects outweigh the supposed benefits; know that you can already get all the benefits met by engaging in other healthy activities that will declutter your mind and liberate you spiritually. Lastly, on this note, in anything, if the bad is more than the good, then it is worth thinking that it is something not worth venturing into.

God did save me from the spirit of masturbation. I did repent from this sin and destruction. *You too can be free from sexual immorality if you submit your body to God totally and give your body to God as a sacrifice for sanctification daily.*

◎ Social Media ◉

You cannot be with everybody at the same time and expect to complete your tasks at the set time. On the one hand, you can sacrifice your social life and gain time sowing it into creativity, which would lead to productivity, so you can show what you have done with your time. On the other hand, you can have a very good social life, but at the end of the year, you have no seeds as proof of how incredibly your time has been spent.

I began to draw myself back from the world of social media slowly before I heard God's instruction in 2020 to not make myself common online; then I gradually removed myself from certain platforms that I was shown not to post on. Social media is addictive, and anything that one is addicted to that makes them devote all their precious time into it is a kind of abuse. So a million people are abusing themselves online and know it not as well as being exploited by the site owners, who know it.

Here is a reflection of me then when I was fascinated by social media. I remember once not having an appetite for food because of the exhaustion built up on my body and mind because of the hours I had spent online. I could see myself cheating myself by spending hours on social media, going from one page to another, when I should have been writing page by page of my book. So I thought, 'What business do I have on social media platforms when I should face my own book?' The more I thought of this metaphor, the closer I was pressed to pen my thoughts and experiences.

Paraphrasing what he preached about the Holy Spirit, talking of the person of the Holy Spirit, Pastor Ayo uses an illustration to emphasise that our identity is in the Holy Ghost. He says that the images we spend time posting on social media are not our real selves. He begins by saying that if we have not begun our journey as believers with the Holy Spirit, then we have not yet begun our journey as believers in general.

Our real person aligns with the Holy Spirit as it is fixed with our mentality, and our mentality is who we really are, not the images we post on social media.

— Pastor Ayodeji Ajibulu, Living Faith Surrey International

Speaking of social media, I learned the hard way that obedience is better than sacrifice. I went back to God in 2020 to ask for permission so that I could post my pictures on social media after I had been instructed clearly not to; when He tells me to and where He points me to, then shall I go. As we know, there are evil eyes all over the world, and they live mostly on the Internet. So when God is telling us, 'No. Not yet. Not here. There,' we should learn to trust His guidance and follow His lead. Therefore, until He announces us to the world, we should keep on advertising Him to our world.

◎ Communication ◉

Listening is the key ingredient for any form of interactive communication, even that with the self and when communicating with GOD and others. You know, there are a lot of conversations that happen in our heads and are communicated back to our minds before we accept or reject them in our hearts. ***Whatever we accept to remain in our heart flows to the rest of our body.***

When it comes to communication from my work supervision feedback, many other sources have told me that my communication skills are very good. Still, I know and have come to realise that I have to work a great deal on my skills in the area of listening to hear those who are the nearest to me because when it comes to talking to my nearest and dearest, I find it a reaction that needs a give-and-take response.

There is a saying: **'It's those who are close to you who will tell you that your mouth needs toothpaste.'** I have been told from time to time by my dearest to 'listen', and I have had to hear them because it is not about me when someone comes to pour their heart out; no matter how tempting it is to think that speaking will solve everything, sometimes just listening will make everything sort itself out. When we are too quick to speak, we miss the point they are trying to express, and so we fail to sieve out the sand from the soul so that the emotional support that they need would be concentrated on. If they are a young person, when this happens, we run the risk of pushing them outdoors to cry on the shoulders of those who may not share the same spiritual and moral sense as we do, which could complicate issues at home or make the young person close up.

Another aspect of communication that frustrates conversations is when one party keeps interrupting the other. It can be very intimidating to be spoken over repeatedly, especially when the dominating partner does not have a sense of awareness that the conversation is not a one-way but a two-way conversation. Speaking too fast soon after someone has made a statement can embarrassingly lead to commenting on non-related subject if we are not paying attention in the first instance. During incidents like these, when it happens in a conversation, whatever the less dominating candidate brings to the table can easily be disregarded, which can make them feel dejected.

When you are too quick to speak before the other person finishes their speech, you bring them into a halt, failing to realise that they were still talking. It's not really of importance to be so quick to suggest a solution or offer advice because most times, we as a people are only just looking for someone to listen to us and feel heard. Sometimes they don't even need an answer; they just want to vent; although the questions they ask are rhetorical and they have the answers, they need acceptance, not dismissal or ignorance.

Effective listening is not ignoring. It will be eventually obvious to whoever is being ignored that they are being ignored. It is better not to engage in a conversation with a person rather than to ignore them and kill their morale by ignoring them. Rather than do that, unintentionally or not, it is better to rebook or refer them to who can better talk with them if you feel that you are not the right person for them to talk to.

Talking is a very sensitive aspect of our lives as people come into it with emotions and energy. Another risk when we don't offer our ears to our nearest and dearest is that because our minds may be too busy cooking up a reply, we may become judgemental and offensive knowingly or unknowingly.

◯ **Writing** ⊛

Finding the right time to write as well as finding the right space to write, for me, is very important because the focus has to be kept on the inspirations in passing so that they can be captured with a net. Separating what inspirations I need for this book project from what inspirations I need for my other projects without losing track of new inspirations and ideas is a skill that God is still teaching me so that I don't lose focus on the project at hand.

I love writing and enjoy searching out and jotting down the meanings of new or repeated words that I have heard either from the mouths of men or from the voice of God. When I was a little girl, I used to write stories and hide them under my mattress. I felt that my handwriting was so bad that I thought if I could not read it, how was it possible that anyone else could? I still remember the times when I joked about writing with my left feet, which was why it was bad (LOL), but I know better now than to put myself down, not even in jokes as jokes carry almost 100 per cent of truth in them.

In the year 2020, God did something I never knew would happen in a hurry. Shortly after I began to write down the things that the Holy Spirit was both telling and teaching me, I noticed that it came in numbers, so I had to purchase all types of journals so I could keep up with both writing from my private daily studies with God as well as writing down revelations I received during the course of the day and those from reading books and articles by other authors. ***What happened next amazed me. My writing kept getting better and better, from good to better to the best, and I am still growing towards my 'better best' so that I can do my 'greater best'.***

Later on in the year, I wrote two separate notes and delivered them separately to my siblings in July 2020. Their reactions made me understand what God is seriously doing in my life as He is set to take me from glory to glory until the perfect day when Jesus returns.

'Who wrote this?' was the question of one, the other asking, 'Did you write this?'

It was at this moment that I realised my handwriting had gotten from bad to good. I replied to one of my siblings jokingly, 'Yes, I wrote it with anointed fingers.'

They replied, 'I never knew that an adult's writing can change from bad to good in their adult years.'

'This is only what I can do' was my answer, and I was praying to God to bring this conversation to a close so that it was obvious whom all the glory should go to.

I used to ask members of my household to help me write out my roughly handwritten messages on my behalf to avoid being laughed at. This was how I could not be surprised at the reactions of my siblings because everybody knew me as the weakest link in the house until I got into Christ; now people who knew me before ask if this is the real me. ***The real me is in Christ, who made me a wonder to the world through His marvellous works in my life.***

Typing what I have written is easier when I can read what I have written. So I am really grateful to God for making my writing come round. I learned how to type back in school; I can still see the image of me and my former schoolmates Carol, Godfrey, Minyen, and Kuvinda as well as the rest of us laughing at our computer teacher for teaching us how to type, along with Zoe and those who took it seriously. Little did I know that the skills learned then are helping me to type rather well today.

I am aware that there are other quicker ways of typing, such as speaking into the device for the words to appear on the screen. As for me, typing has been very therapeutic for me. It has also been a rewarding experience for me to see my achievements go from penned to typewritten, printed, and published; this gives me courage that I can do more through Christ if I put my mind to it.

Learning how to type, we laughed at our teachers then, but today we find the skills they taught us still important, making no knowledge wasted, and we know that the right knowledge is key to avoiding a wasted life.

◯ Reading ◉

The books I read in 2020 were not as many as I had listed down at the beginning of this year because of certain distractions that were out of this world but forced their way into my life. Luckily, I began reading at the start of the year so I could retain a reframing mentality from the contents I'd gained before the challenges came. I read some books in the Bible and studied some characters from the Bible. I, however, noticed that sometimes when I would pick up something to read, the Holy Spirit would direct me to read something else or would place a scripture in my heart for me to revisit.

Sometimes, to be honest, I'd never heard of most of the things God told me first but found them in the Bible. Some of the scriptures the Holy Ghost deposited into my spirit (but not all) include **Amos 3:3**. In the passage is a simple question of whether two can work together except agree; it carries great wisdom when one approaches a given situation with this question in mind, especially when it comes to relationships with other people, which are in everything we do because we build our lives and businesses around people, and God is always sending us to people.

There are a few others, but I did wonder 'What is it that God is showing me here?' so that I could look more closely into it and think deeply into my own life and whether I am on track with His plan for my life. Some books I read in 2020 are the following:

- *Anointing for Exploits* **by David O. Oyedepo**
- *Pillars of Destiny (The 12 Pillars of Destiny)* **by David O. Oyedepo**

When I read these books, God spoke to me in volumes to the extent that I began to look for hills in my community to run up. Stan saw this and got mad because each time I ran, I did what I could not do. I did not stop at that but voiced out, 'Thank you, Jesus! I have broken limits with a supernatural and drastic shift!' without knowing that the devil was calculating how to trip me up. MY LORD Jesus was making me skip through mountains in the supernatural realm that were backed up with prophetic words from Bishop David Oyedepo and Apostle Paul Eneche, as spoken by God through their mouths.

- *Satan, Get Lost: Outstanding Breakthroughs* **by David O. Oyedepo**

The testimonies in *Satan, Get Lost* gave me hope that I would surely testify. I read *Satan, Get Lost* some years back but followed the direction of Pastor Nicolas Udoh of Living Faith Canaanland to reread this book, coupled with fasting. I must have read this book for the fourth time in a short space of time. Sometimes I read it chapter by chapter each day; other days, I read it in chunks of pages per period. Following reading strategies like this so that I would not be overwhelmed with other activities really took away the pressure from my shoulders, which allowed the pleasure of reading to rest on me.

What is important about reading books again, particularly when in the middle of a war, is that your intellect may have seen the words, but your spirit is still waiting to cite the word so that your spirit and the spirit of God can spark before the light comes on to turn off the darkness that is resisting for the battle to be prolonged.

- ***Supernatural Childbirth* by Jackie Mize**

Rereading *Supernatural Childbirth* by Jackie Mize helped me rebuild my faith in God to affirm that I am serving a God of miracles.

- ***Withstanding the Devil* by Watchman Nee**

Withstanding the Devil showed me how tricky yet weak the devil becomes when you resist him and take authority over him. I miraculously meet Cassie online via an invitation in my email during the lockdown. I know Cassie applauded my reading collection in 2020. I recall telling her that I believed my reading should be more than I did, and I really thought so without trying to impress anyone. If anything, be inspired instead because it is said that **'readers are leaders'**, right?

Cassie maintained a weekly hour-long call for our prayer and discussion of the word of God. At the interval of our gathering, Cassie suddenly told me that she picked up a book for me as a gift, but I did not get to find out what the name of the book was until it arrived through the Royal Mail post. Without knowing what God was preparing me for, I gladly received and read the book as soon as I opened it.

When I was discussing aspects of the book that I liked with Cassie, Cassie informed me that she'd had two choices, but she chose to buy *Withstanding the Devil* for me without knowing that she was working with God to prepare me for the road ahead; she remained in obedience to the lead of the Holy Spirit.

Withstanding the Devil talks strongly about resisting the devil. I recall making some interesting notes and feeling empowered during my read. Shortly after I was blessed with this book and reading it, I was attacked in a battle in an extreme manner, so much so that only took the mercy of God to make me survive the war.

- ### *My Mental Health Matter: Beginnings* by Merisha Meisha

God is so wonderful. I wrote this book. Towards what I call the end of the book in November 2020, the enemy broke out with a war in my head to force me out from my divine project. However, I refused to give up because I saw the hands of God always with me, so I began to read *Beginnings*, and it just kept me on God's flow, which enabled me to keep flowing with the will of God in my life.

This book spoke to me like it's speaking to you now, and it became the rope that God used to pull me out from the waters where my enemies thought I would remain. Generally, I enjoy reading and wish to create secluded time for reading apart from the Bible. I am also happy to learn of how much happiness and encounters can come from reading. I say this especially because it is an area I have shied away from in my past because of a deceptive impression of myself as dyslexic.

The Mask

COVID-19 is the MASK that demons used to dispatch their evil operations in the darkest time of a year full of blood. The number of people who have died from the coronavirus is incredible, but more incredible is the number of people who do not see the need for salvation and think that it is normal to remain normal in our relationship with God.

Haba! Coronavirus restrictions saw intensive hospital screening, which meant the majority of people with other illnesses and sicknesses were not allowed hospital admission. The hospital, which is a place for treatment, could not allow all who were sick in because of the coronavirus precautions that were in practice. On the other hand, the place of healing, which is the church, was not allowed to be open, so the church doors were closed to those who needed to be desperately well.

A zillion demons that were released from hell in 2020 found their ways into the community of living people they wanted dead. True, most people feared whatever this COVID-19 was all about and ran to God, while others were kept away from God by the fear of not trusting an invisible God as if COVID-19 had not come as a sign of waning that not all will be seen but must be felt at one time or another.

In the year 2021, a lot of people are still walking around with anxiousness on the effect of the coronavirus, some of whom were affected directly and others who were affected indirectly. The populous citizens of the world had to change the way they lived and related with themselves and others as a result of the coronavirus. I have heard people say, 'Even after COVID-19, I'm still gonna wear my mask.' The coronavirus has left so much ambiguity in the lives of millions in my community to the extent where fear has almost taken a fixed position in the hearts of men.

An example of how fear controls the thoughts and behaviour of a person after a traumatic event is seen with Mikel. I met Mikel on the train in July 2021 while she was on her way to work. Mikel works in the DLR, stating, 'I have been vaccinated, and I have my mask on, so I am safe.' This was a great conversation starter, I noticed, and she started it, so it suggested to me that Mikel had more that she may want to get off her chest, and her body language indicated so. So I wanted to hear her.

The short of it is that she is an American who lives in Britain. Her buoyant self stemmed from her being American, I observed, but even underneath her buoyant attitude and brave character, she was afraid, and I could see this unease in the middle and lower sides of her body. There was heaviness on her chest and tension in her curled toes. Mikel caught COVID-19 and was treated for the virus in 2020, so she was being obviously careful, but unknowing to her, she was walking in the fear of being overly cautious so as not to catch the virus again.

It was interesting to see Mikel's breathing go from erratic to steady when I mentioned that God was my source of safety – not undermining her experience. Mikel became more conversational and added that God was the author of her life and that it was He who had used her experience to prepare her for her managerial work with the homeless team project in the United Kingdom. **POWERFUL.**

Our experience either makes us experience fright or fight. If we refuse to experience fright, it makes us fly to high heights. This mask called COVID-19 came to steal hope, time, destinies, and lives, but know that you are a survivor of it. Note though that the most important thing of being a survivor of COVID-19 is knowing that you survived COVID-19 for a reason. There is a reason why God spared your life, so don't forget to show your gratitude to God and, in your appreciation, ask Him, 'Why are you here still?' so that you can walk into His plan for you now rather than later.

Living is not going to work and paying the bills; if this is all it is, this is depression. Living is staying in God's purposed plan for your life; this is the vision for living. COVID-19 has done so much damage to mankind, but the lessons that it has taught us should never be taken for granted. There are teenagers who lost proper education and experienced all kinds of hardship that they had not dealt with in their lives. COVID-19 is not selective with age, gender, or race; it affects all, but this unique experience should pull us together as a people, and we should still look up to God for a solution. The world needs God's intervention to deal with the destruction that is happening in different parts of the world. The dominating news of COVID-19 (masking up and preventing it) stay in the limelight. For example, news hardly spread of the massacres/killings happening in the populous villages, towns, and cities of Nigeria on a daily basis.

◯ **Sleeping Time** ◉

Don't be scared when you wake up in the early hours of the morning. It does not matter if you are the only one in your home who is used to waking up in the early hours of the day. Just like everyone's lifestyle is different, so are our relationships with God. So submitting yourself to God early is beneficial for your spiritual growth. The early hours are the time of spiritual warfare, so be alert and allow God to use you to quench the altars of dark and evil powers with the fire of the Holy Ghost burning in your heart and pouring out from your prayers.

Sleep is a gift from God, and only He has the authentication to wake us up in the morning. Even though we can decide what time we go to bed, we can never decide to wake ourselves up without the help of God, regardless of the function of an alarm clock. I have heard Pastor Nathaniel Odin of Living Faith International say, 'If it was the alarm clock that woke us up, then why not place the alarm clock in the mortuary and count how many dead persons will come back to life as soon as the alarm sets off?'

I like having enough rest when I go to bed so that by the time I get up from bed, I feel well rested and energised for the day's activities ahead. However, waking up early is part of my routine, although the time varies. Still, without the aid of an alarm clock lately and purely by a tap from the Holy Ghost, I am awoken into the new dawn for a brand new season each day.

When I wake up early, I give thanks to God for making me a number among the living on earth and not with the dead in the grave. Waking up early before everyone else also gives me that advantage overall because I use my time to devote some time alone with the Holy Spirit, separate from everything else, before the rest of the world gets up and becomes busy with their business. In addition, one of the reasons I enjoy coming before God first thing in the morning is that after this, I get renewed inspiration and so become more productive and accomplish a lot more than I set out for myself in the day should I have started a different way. *So in other words, it is time spent but time also gained, coming before God at the beginning of the day.*

Lastly, I do not feel guilty for devoting my hours to God at such hours at the beginning of the day because during the course of the day, I do not underachieve; I do not feel tired or feel like I need a coffee to stay up. *I never drink coffee for any occasion but yet am energised by the strength of GOD.* In due course, I achieve more when I wake up early because after I have finished my devotion and studies, I do my exercise, and when I have completed my activities and morning routine, I feel ready to resume work; this is when I hear the world waking up.

I hear God's voice louder early in the morning. So I give God the best part of me in the early hours of the day, which, in turn, equally sees the best of me come out. I make God the God over my life by submitting myself to Him first thing in the morning so that even my thanksgiving and gratitude to God in this part of the day are more authentic than usual, as if the beginning of the day is not already crowded with turbulence or noise from the busyness of the day. *On the whole, my praise and singing are on similar frequencies as those of birds tweeting at this time of the day.*

◐ Insomnia ◑

Did you know that both physical and mental health conditions are medical health concerns and conditions and that insomnia falls under mental health conditions, whether it is diagnosed or not? So let's stop the stigma already and get healed quickly.

You roll into the night as daylight steals your sleep; still, your light refuses to switch off in your mind's eye. He never stops hearing the clock tick over his head, laid under the pillow. You hear him screaming, 'You devil!' daily as he wakes up without a rise but thinks it early. I say, 'Insomnia, get lost!'

Sleeping to rest the body is a beautiful thing and a gift from the Most High God.

On 13 February 2021. I was invited by Mercy D. from Royal Borough Greenwich London as a guest speaker in the black, Asian, and minority ethnic (BAME) community for a well-being discussion that engaged the power of the mind in the COVID-19 period. The discussion was held on Zoom and hosted by Stella N. from the Faith and Health Promotion Association.

Among other things, I talked about my sleeping habits during COVID-19 because for a whole month in 2020, from May to June, I experienced 'insomnia'. To this day, it is the darkest trick the devil has ever played on me, but thanks to God, I found a switch, and God got me out of that darkness into His light by restoring my sleep to eternity.

As shown below, I have gone ahead and included my notes on that day for the subject I spoke about.

(One)

Introduction

I use therapeutic and creative intervention, along with my spiritual belief, to tackle and nourish my mental health as well as coach others into wellness.

The person who originally recommended for me to share my experiences and work with my community was my medical doctor, who suggested that I begin sharing my experience with normal people who have experienced anxiety. He also suggested that I extend this to people who experience other mental health–related issues to help them progress, having heard what I'd done that helped me progress from ill mental health to a sound mind. However, the supernatural being who empowered me to talk about and share these experiences is the person of the Holy Spirit.

My doctor was moved to have this discussion with me since he noticed the improvement in both my physical and mental health soon after I began to engage my spiritual practices as a method for my healing. Practicing these interventions consistently has resulted in the advancement of my health and general well-being.

I have worked with Mercy in the past, another guest speaker and co-organiser who recommended me as a guest speaker in this panel. Today I am bringing with me to this session my very own experiences and extensive observations and involvements of the world around me.

Currently, I am working with a family providing emotional support for a mother who needs help to manage anxiety as well as supporting this mother with what she is already doing to assist her child, who has some underlying health issues triggered by some psychological factors still under debate.

When you hear the saying 'mental health', what is the first thing that runs through your MIND? Don't answer! Allow the question to sit in your mind for now.

This discussion is based on the power of the mind. Below is how I engaged my mind in the COVID-19 pandemic season to enhance my mental health/well-being. The topic I'm bringing into this subject is on **SLEEP** because even the creator of heaven and earth rested on the seventh day of His creation.

One area I noticed when I decided to take charge of my own mental health/well-being was that thinking of what other people say stopped me from doing what I wanted to do publically. In other words, it disabled certain movements that could have led to improvement in my life. This pushed me to begin to do things so differently.

For example, when I want to dance in the snow – outdoors, of course – with the intention of using this as a way of expressing my happiness, I stop thinking of what people are thinking because I know that if they could be as brave as me or could let out the child in them, they would probably want to do what I am doing if they don't think about what other people would think of them.

(Two)

Relaxing the Mind

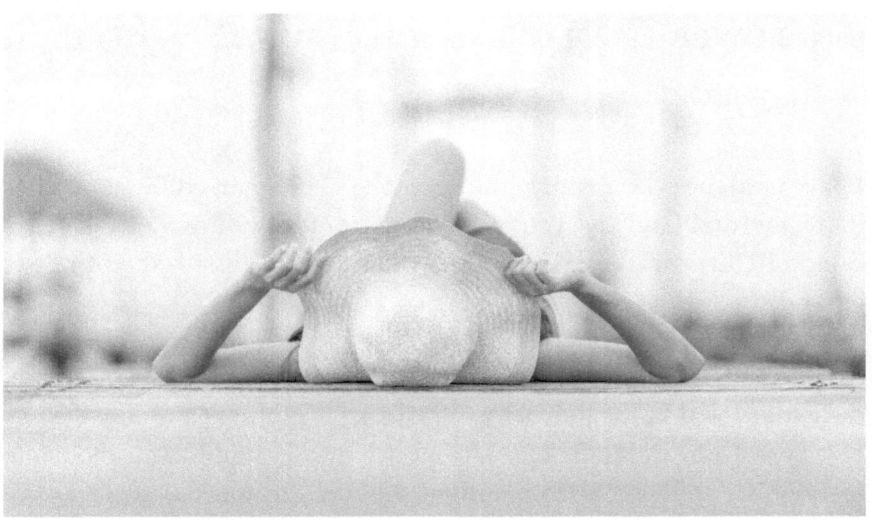

Close your eyes for a minute if you are comfortable to do so. Then smile to relax your muscles while you think of nothing for a minute. Mummy Elephant asked for just five minutes of peace for those who are familiar with the book by Jill Murphy titled *Five Minutes' Peace*.

If you had five minutes to yourself today, what would you do with your five minutes? Take a minute to pause.

(Three)

When the Mind Says 'Go'

It takes quite a lot of dedication to move the mind to act upon what you want to see change. However, first, you must make the decision of wanting the changes you want to see happen. Then apply consistency in your application of the change you want to see manifest.

I know that it's not child's play when it comes to using the power of the mind to defeat and overcome frightful and difficult happenings, but I have decided to choose faith over fear in such difficult times as COVID-19. In doing so, I daily subscribe to the word of the almighty God, my creator, who said to me, 'I have not given you the spirit of fear but of **POWER** and of **LOVE** and a sound **MIND**.'

POWERFUL.

I have used the power of my mind to engage in so many different battles in my life, and God has won recent fights for me because I engaged the mind of Christ in the midst of it all, fully involved with the mind-set of God.

'When the Mind Says "Go"' is a poem I wrote centred on a very difficult period in the journey of my life that captures a different story of where I am today in life. However, what is significant about me mentioning this is that to highlight the force in movement when we engage the power of our minds to move forward, it pushes us further to swim across the deep ends.

WHEN THE MIND SAY GO

BY MEISHA MERISHA

HEAD MIND AND LEGS
THE HEAD IS FULL
WHEN THE BODY SAYS GO
THE LEGS GETS WEAKEN BY THE KNEE
WHEN THE HEART SAYS GO
THE HANDS ARE SHAKEN LIKE A LEAF
BUT WHEN THE MIND SAYS GO
IS TIME TO STOMACH ALL AND MOVE

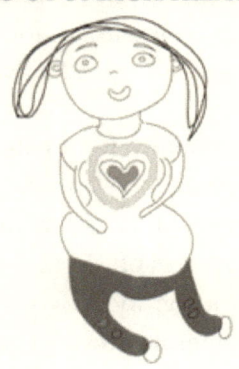

October 2013 Artist life performance

My Mental Health Matters

(Four)

<u>Mindful Sleep</u>

Sleeping and waking up adds a good reason to live life, while sleeping and not waking up is said to be death. As sleep happens to be an important factor of life, the majority of people don't get enough sleep to help them live longer and healthier these days, especially with the younger generation nowadays.

Sleep is as natural as nature itself. In essence, give sleep a chance to rest your body and allow sleep to happen when it comes instead of fighting if off. As common as it may sound (because it happens every day), when sleep stops happening as a daily recurrence, I say this could either mean living a dead life or living life in a deadly manner.

What is sleep, and why is sleep important to me? I tried to find out what sleep means to me, and I discovered that when I don't have enough sleep, I cannot function properly in the daytime. This is because my brain gets tired, having been put to work for the best hours in the course of the day. As a result, my mind is not as sound as it should be to empower the rest of my body to be productive profoundly.

Sleep is said to contribute majorly to our living, apart from food and other essentials like water. Sleep is the foundation created for the body to sit comfortably while allowing other pillars that move the body around to build up the person. If we stave off sleep, sleep will deprive our bodies from rest when they need it the most. My sleep time and how many hours of sleep I need to recuperate are personal to me depending on my lifestyle; this is to say that sleep happens uniquely to each individual, and there is no set time to sleep and wake up. However, I found out that the best sleep is at night because of the quietness of the night, and naturally, sleep is designed for the night, when the daylight is gone.

Jesus Christ said in John 9:4 after healing the man who was born blind that He must work in the daytime, for the night time comes where no one man can work. What this means for me is that day and night are designed for their specific reasons and that the activities that they host are best performed in the time they are set out to be carried out in. Saying this, I understand that most people work at night, especially in European countries, so when sleep happens, makes the most of it.

No matter what time I climb onto my bed, when my brain switches off, that's when sleep happens to me. Still, I find it interesting that our minds can still be active when the brain has gone to rest. This does not mean that a busy mind is a healthy mind because when the mind is overworked, the mind's eyes can refuse to be shut, therefore causing insomnia to occur.

Insomnia, in description, occurs in this form: even when you are tired yet, you can't fall deep into sleep. You lie with your eyes closed all night for hours, but when you open them, you feel like you haven't shut them all throughout the night. This is because the body has not produced enough chemicals to make you sleepy. So you spend the day exhausted and sometimes even yawning but still can't get shuteye.

The reason why a person cannot fall asleep even when their body demands it excessively is because the pineal gland produces the melatonin hormone, which is responsible for making one sleepy, and this is mixed with the norepinephrine hormone, which makes a human sleepy and fall asleep when the two are mixed together.

Constant deprivation of sleep will eventually affect the performance of the brain and mind-set of a person, which can lead to tiredness; there could be slight but noticeable dysfunctions in the person's life.

Now tiredness could lead to so many things, including making mistakes. In so doing, this may lead to triggering other underlying mental health issues in the person, such as signs of nervousness. When a person is nervous over a certain period, this could lead to anxiety. Anxiety, if not taken care of, can lead to the deterioration of one's mental health.

Did you know that a majority of the people who suffer from insomnia in black communities are those who work at night?

Another category of people who suffer from insomnia apart from the youth is young children who have suffered or are still suffering from abuse, especially sexual abuse because they are scared that the attackers/abusers will come back to attack them at any given time unannounced. Women whose husbands usually rape them while they are asleep can adequately be too afraid to fall asleep naturally, so as a mechanism to guide them, they keep themselves up initially, but as this pattern of fear is prolonged, it graduates to insomnia, unfortunately. Most young people, especially in England, suffer from insomnia, so to aid their sleep, they resort to drug abuse.

My Sleep in COVID-19 2020

In the year of COVID-19, between May and June 2020, I noticed a sudden but major shift in my sleep pattern that left me sleepless for fourteen nights straight. This is one of the scariest ordeals that I have ever experienced in my lifetime. It seemed like it had happened all of a sudden, but it was a gradual build-up until the day it actually happened.

On that faithful evening, I had gone to bed and closed my eyes as usual, hoping to fall asleep as I do, but my beauty sleep was taken away from my eyes because it had gone out my mind. I am known as 'Sleeping Beauty' by my friend Idalina, and people who know me well already know that when I go to bed, I create such an atmosphere that prevents me from being bothered by anything. So it was odd for them to hear me say sleep had not happened.

However, for the first time in my life, I truly could empathise with the people who are unable to sleep for whatever reason. I also truly knew what they meant when they said, 'I can't sleep.' I used to think it was like not being able to sleep throughout the night but at least for some hours. Not in my wildest dream had I never thought that it meant as they said until I could not sleep for two weeks straight.

Do you know that when you sleep, your mind is still active?
Who did it happen to? This happened to me. I was incredibly creative during the first part of the lockdown, and so was my mind, at work constantly even after I left my desk. I have such a creative mind, so when I opened up that part of my psyche, my mind's eye lit up, as bright as a fluorescent light, and I'd only learned that this was the case after three nights of not being able to sleep. What I did do to gain back sleep was I had my first conversation with God about this because He gives His beloved sleep so that they can use their daytime for work and night time for resting.

Did you know that insomnia is a mental health illness? The next best thing I did was pick up the phone and call a few people I knew who had already described these sleepless nights to me as an issue they were experiencing in their lives. I called and **reasoned with and reassured** them that I knew how it felt to be in such dark place. Because I was trying different methods, I discussed my application with them so that they too could tap into it for their healing through my methods. Using the word of faith, I found helpful to keep myself away from fear. I changed my sleeping position and changed my bedtime and room lighting as well as my room temperature.

However, my sleep was only restored when I began to give praise to God in the middle of the night when I could not sleep. This was what had worked for me and for God. To prove that my miracle was certain, I was minding my own business one day when a woman I had met at church called me up and said she could not sleep for days. Even if my body was tense and I could not think my way out of my sleepless nights, I used the power of my mind to reinforce my belief that with God, all things are possible.

It took me engaging in the power of my mind to believe God for a miracle because I have heard people say that they have not been able to sleep for up to six years in some instances. Saying so, I knew my miracle was granted the second I received a text message with an invitation to pray for this person who was unable to sleep as a long-term mental health problem. I quickly ran to her house to pray with her, and we did pray with her daughter in their garden because we were still in lockdown.

(Five)

Let's Talk About Mental Health

My mental health matters to 'who', 'what', 'when', 'where', and 'why'. Most people may still be too shy to openly talk about their mental health concerns. I believe the reason behind this conspicuous way of relating to the term 'mental health' is due to the lack of understanding what it is and the lack of awareness of what it is about, especially in some African countries that are still too adamant to accept that the collapse of someone's mental health could be a result of either psychological or spiritual affliction to one's mental health. Embracing the matter of the incident when a person's mental health deteriorates is not as simple as blaming the condition as a result of the suffering individual coming down with a mental health illness because of what he/she or their parents may have done in the past and so forth.

Most governmental systems around the world that are dismissive of this subject, mental health, and that are reluctant to convey funding in this sector are seeing fast-disappearing young Africans abuse drugs and end up contemplating suicide because of the oppressive government systems in Africa that are exploiting citizens and denying the people their basic human rights.

Most often, these governments are dismissive because they themselves do not know enough about the subject and so are incapable of making good judgements of sound mind. I say this because a sound mind will not lead people into debt, dismay, disillusion, and detriment, which have forced millions of youths into prostitution and drug abuse, which is, in itself, a mental health disorder – the fact that the drug is needed as a substitute to perform what the body should naturally do.

Mental health facilities are generally underestimated in most nations across the world, which give more emphasis on facilities for physical health. Mental health has depth and so much elements to it, yet you don't have separate clinics for each of the categories, as is the case in physical health. Thus, mental health facilities still lack medical attention because of the way the issue is grouped categorically with some of its conditions.

Governments and individuals who lack awareness of what mental health really is and the importance of taking care of their mental health will really struggle to seek help in this area of their lives if needed and so will not know what department to go to for help if needed. In addition, there is a fear that mounts up for some when they hear the term 'mental health', so it needs to be broken down to some people so that they can accept help and prayers when they are called for.

Moving forward on this matter, mental health, simply termed, is 'brain health'. I think we should find ways to break it down to terms that we are comfortable to embrace, which would allow us to nurture our mental health in better ways rather than writing endless reports on budget demands win Africa. Needs must go straight to the people who matter in the community by going to them, finding out what their needs are, and then setting up hubs in the community, like drop-ins with trained staff and reachable staff where the local people can go to for help when it's needed.

At the initial stage of COVID-19, many people thought COVID-19 was just a fluke and not the flu. They also thought that it would soon fly away, but it stayed and lingered longer than anticipated. In its duration, it changed the way we receive one another and how we protect ourselves from one another in ways never seen since the beginning of our creation and existence. The pandemic has changed our behaviours and thought patterns, which all originate from the mind.

'Hungry London' is a poem that is the summary of how I found myself in my neighbourhood and where I taught my mind to be in my body, an expression of where I had been with myself at the time I wrote the poem. *'Hungry London'* also allowed me to see myself when the world was taken away from me as well as people kept far away from themselves and the world kept far away from itself.

I shared my poem 'Hungry London' with the audience. This was selected by Pen to Print as one of the best poems in 2020, which was published in their magazine *Write On*. The poem is below. I thank the person who read it out for the audience.

Hungry London

Poem by Meisha Merisha

Have you thought of me since I walked pass your house
hungry
Do you recognize my face under your mask when you
peek into my eyes
Can you tell I observed you quickly crossing over the road
with two Tesco bags
Did you notice I opened my mouth to say you a hello' but
closed it up gain at once
Would you mind the gap if I stood on the edge of the
pavement
Could you tell I waited for you to walk on by as you do
and you did
Did you see me wear a smile when you wore your gloves
with a frown
Not a blink or a wave; still I'm famished, I saw you vanished in rampage for
food
Was I on your mind when you closed your doors and left me panting on your
doormat like a baby fox wondering where's everybody
Can you see me standing here naked; Posed vampish but dampish hair on
silky skin
How cold I felt, did you feel? As you hastily swiped my skin in grab for
tissues
Is it easy to spot the goosebumps on my body; not because I tremble from the
frost, but because you snatched the frozen seeded bread I held so close to my
chest with thoughts to feed the birds of the streets
Can you sense I seek to hide my face in the curve of my palm when I saw you
sanitize your hands after meeting my body with yours in your grab for bread
Still you keep the bread happily away form the birds
While I keep my smile till June allure of a sunny day in loop for the news
shopper
Will I not cry in wonder of such a solitary mews where there should be
solidarity in a time of uncertainty; I gaze up to heaven for my rainbow;
When you are locked in
eating, and I'm locked out twirling with the birds tweeting, I'll be the
rainbow in your cloud.

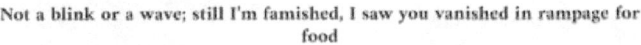

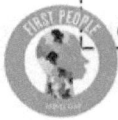

 My Mental Health Matters

A one-minute exercise is done to emphasise that in our busyness, we should give our minds more than a minute of silence and spend some peaceful time alone to reflect and be grateful to God for how we got to where we are in one piece, even in the midst of the stormy season.

- Was it possible to think about nothing for a minute?
- Were you able to think about nothing for a minute?
- What did you notice you were anxious about when you tried thinking about nothing for a minute?
- What was persistently coming back to your mind when you tried thinking about nothing for a minute?
- Can you recall your heart rate when you tried thinking about nothing for a minute?
- When you were thinking about nothing for a minute, did you notice any tone of voice coming to your mind?
- When you were thinking about nothing for a minute, the voice that you noticed, having identified the tone or whether you did or did not hear a voice – was it from your spirit or the spirit of God?

Answers to Questions

I can share an example of how to use the power of the mind to mend your mind; this has helped me remain focused on my activity and kept me engaged in a gainful activity, such as exercising. I drew out this idea during my exercise on the snow by being mindful of the voice that began a conversation in my mind. As long as my mind is activated, this is something that happens sporadically, but what I do with the voice is what makes the difference in my mental health.

Now what I mean by 'voices' is not the hearing of voices during a psychosis episode, such as auditory hallucinations. The voices described above are conversations in one's head that happen to everyone all the time when they are trying to finish a conversation that is cut short or trying to process new information or a new idea that pops into their mind.

One day it snowed, the first day of the snow. I woke up to see the pretty white streets, but this did not deter me from my routine. The snow made me not want to run because I did not want to fall down, so I decided to dance on the ice instead.

Now it may look crazy to other people, but I was keeping safe and keeping fit at the same time because my mind was like 'If I run, I will fall, but if I go back indoors, I have not fulfilled the purpose of taking myself outdoors'. To win this battle in my mind, I trained my mind not to see anyone else but myself on the ice because even if people may think that I look stupid for dancing on the ice, I know that I am doing something extra that will enhance my mental health/well-being.

I made a point of doing this because many times, it is easy to forget that by taking care of our physical health, we are helping our mental health not deteriorate. What helped me engage my mind to remain focused was not to pay attention to the voices that rose up in my thoughts; a lot of it stemmed from fear.

Fear says, 'You will fall down flat on your face. The ground is horribly slippery, and everyone will laugh at you.'

Faith says, 'You can do anything through your saviour, who will lift you up even if you fall.'

Choosing faith over fear is what brings on my confidence as the picture changes, and as soon as I begin to see the images in my mind, as my saviour says it, the lioness in me comes alive and empowers my mind to move and reach for the mountaintops. Even if I don't get to the top at once, I have begun the process, and as long as I stay in the process, the lifting occurs naturally. This is because each time I try, I am empowered to try again because of the satisfaction gained from previous attempts, and I go on and on until the completion of my task. Still, the key ingredient is consistency. This is what fuels the mind to remain powerful to take on faith over fear.

Thank you.

◯ Coaching You through Wellness ◉

These are the author's responses to some of the questions asked about herself and the book.

Please tell us a little about yourself, Merisha.

I'm a beautiful personality with a very creative and sound mind. I am a well-being mentor with experience in working in special needs education as a wellness support worker with children and family outside the classroom environment. Other times, I have worked as a teaching assistant within the classroom setting. Apart from my work in special needs education, I am a mental health advocate and an author. Although my journals are mainly thought-provoking in the mental health sector, they draw out how I have used my faith to overcome life challenges.

I have been told by tutors that I am resilient and by my supervisors that I am dedicated. For the people I have helped, I have often been told that I am very supportive even when providing emotional support to them, which comes naturally to me. Other people have said that I have a strong character, but I know it is because I have a powerful God backing me up in spite of my struggles.

You currently work as a mental wellness coach. When and how did you begin this line of work? What attracted you to this type of work?

I began to take an interest in the mental health sector in 2012, but I did not begin my work in this field until 2014. I got rather passionate about this field of work in 2013 during my studies in therapeutic arts and education. What attracted me to this line of work is seeking answers to some unanswered questions in my own and my family's mental health status.

Tell us what you have been able to do in this field of endeavour, what challenges you have had to deal with, and how you have had to re-invent yourself to stay on track.

This book project is something I have worked on massively since the 2020 global lockdown. This mailing consists of the ministry aspect of my projects and forms a larger part of the My Mental Health Matter project also. Consistently talking about mental health awareness and how to best to care for one's mental well-being is the larger part of my written journal and actual work on the field. For the business aspect of this project, First People Mind Gap have designed some T-shirts to highlight the subject of mental health so as to enhance people's understanding on this topic. The aim of this is to provide an education platform and workshop sections to raise even more awareness on mental health in the community.

I already have a few poems which will be included in some pages of this book. I have also been working on some videos which are ready to go on the website, and again, the images are channelled to help people realise that it is OK to, first, recognise that they have mental health issues and, second, know what they are, which leads to, third, searching and knowing how best to address them.

A few identified challenges are seen in the time I consumed planning before taking up a new task; I noticed the way my brain processes information, although I would not call it time wasted but constructively spent planning so that time is not wasted in the end. Another challenge which has affected the speedy progression of the project is finances of the lack of them. In the past, waiting on the right persons to come on board so we can run the course of the project has also been a factor of delay in essence.

What has helped me stay on track is seeing the vision being painted larger on my mind each day despite the enemy's desperation to see me fall and fail. I receive fresh revelations from God and reflect on the journey so far; how God's grace has brought me this far has kept me inspired and steadfast on the track regardless of hiccups.

Who are the people you work with, and what results have you helped them achieve?

From the angle of my work in ministry, I have been able to pray for some people with various life challenges/issues, especially health concerns, and God almighty has been merciful to send His word quickly to heal them. I have shared some of the testimonies in this book to help them keep looking unto God for their own miracles too. I will say that creating an impact in the lives of the families I have worked with in the community with the work I have been able to do with Greenwich Home Start has brought happiness to me, and I know that I was able to help elevate others. Again, celebrating other people's testimonies via our encounters is God's proof that He is with me.

Most certainly, it's been a joyful experience for me and a thing of joy to be part of other people's joy, but the most significant inspiration of being part of people's journeys is the given grace in lasting in prayer for supplication for God to draw nearer those whom He has healed and equally secure their salvation in Christ Jesus so that their relationship with God will be enhanced.

Did you know you were going to be doing this kind of work at this stage in your life? Is there anything from your childhood that pointed to you doing this work at this stage?

When I was a little girl, my siblings used to tease me for running away from my homework so that I could do the housework. I guess what this says about me from an early age is that I like helping. I was also seen as an interesting kid when I used to run into an empty room and start dancing. I often caught my siblings peeping through the window as I danced.

I see working in the mental health field as a helping, humanitarian role. So if I throw my thoughts back to my early childhood, I would link myself now to my very young self from my primary education years, as far back as I can remember, right through to teenage years and somewhat now. I would say that I have been formed into the person that I was created to become – with personal and spiritual growth, of course.

I also see myself as always looking for people around me to gift with presents, not necessarily materialistic gifts. I reckon that, as mentioned above, I must have been created this way before I could remember myself, in my very early years. My eldest sibling always told me that when I was a very tiny girl, I always shared my food. The events she describes, I don't remember because they go beyond the days of my life that I could remember, but I'm certain she does remember them because there is a good ten years between us.

Saying this, I do remember climbing on top of a stool so I could reach the sink to do the dishes, and I enjoyed tidying the rooms after my siblings and helping around the house, even if my siblings found it funny that I liked cleaning other people's messes rather than exhausted myself in play.

I found your poems intriguing, and I thought I would ask you to share with us your thoughts on the 2020 global lockdown situation as well as issues such as hunger and loneliness arising from that and their impact on mental health. Would you please share your thoughts?

I believe the 2020 lockdown definitely impacted on the mental health/well-being of people all over the world. Locally, I witnessed the radical level of anxiousness in the lives of people, especially young people like teenagers, because their business came to a halt. Some of the activities that teenagers engage themselves in are what they may describe as what keeps them 'seen'. It is also known that they spend large amounts of their time with their friends. So keeping them away from their friends for such a long time as well as insecurity from the lack of income that occurred as a result of job loss during the pandemic certainly raised anxiety among young people because of the restrictions on their expenses and the restricted freedom of movement. Young people already go through a lot of anxiety for the future, although they may not always want to express it because they may feel embarrassed. For others, they may not feel comfortable expressing their feelings because they are used to being judged, so they clam up because they feel they will not be heard.

COVID-19, on the other hand, forced some of the young people I had met and spoken to in my community to admit that the future seemed a bit scary; they did not know what could be round the corner when they were only just starting out in life. Remember, it is already a very scary world for some of these young people because of some of the crimes they witness on the streets; hence, they feel the need to be in groups.

Now I measured the behaviour of many others at the beginning of the lockdown with regard to the 'grab all I can' attitude. They who dived into the stores selfishly did so out of panic, and panic stems from anxiousness because they were most likely nervous about the unknown. Moreover, after the first part of the lockdown, a more calm atmosphere was restored in the community, and I noticed people showing empathy and understanding.

Let's not forget the many homeless and unemployed people who depend on public spaces such as libraries for their social activities; their psychological needs were all forced out, from their comfort zone to Zoom. What about those who are not equipped with electronics and some students who use this public space to complete their assignments?

Among them, there could have been a good number of people who could have been using this public space as a refuge then. So with the doors closed, one can only imagine the high level of anxiety at stake – in the worst case scenario, a detriment for many. COVID-19 arrived unexpectedly without any instant solution, so no one was really prepared for the shock. As such, there are stories in the media of families committing suicide; they unfortunately saw it as a way to escape from it all.

Again, with the lockdown extended into the year, the severity of loneliness is almost inevitable for those people experiencing mild mental health issues and living indecently. They may not fully understand the rules of social distancing and so miss out on daily hour-long exercise opportunities, thereby completely isolating themselves in their houses as a result of public spaces being closed, which will, in turn, make their mental health conditions worse. Furthermore, the general practitioner system changed from face-to-face/manual contact to a digital screen setup system in line with the government's COVID-19 guidelines. This system could certainly increase the patient's anxiety level, especially for the older generation, who are not comfortable with such technology.

However, you have rediscovered purpose during the lockdown. So would you say that adversity always carries a blessing and that perspective is required in overcoming whatever mental health issues threaten to overwhelm us in this season?

I will not say that I rediscovered my purpose during this lockdown because I already got my purpose in life revealed to me by the Holy Spirit before the lockdown, and I began pursuing it. However, the 2020 lockdown, made me run faster because the time that I did not budget for from heaven was downloaded into me.

Saying this, I discovered the importance of pursuing my purpose in life when I did the Winners Chapel Bible School course in 2016–2018, and since then, I have been mindful to stay on track and continue with my creative process.

I would much rather say I had gotten more inspiration during the lockdown, even if the Holy Spirit profoundly revealed my visions to me via revelations before the lockdown. They began to prepare me well in advance; I found ample time in maximising my creativity and building on the technical side of my business.

What is most rewarding about your work? What makes it all worthwhile? As a Christian, what do you bring that is different to the world of mental health?

The most rewarding thing about working in this field is seeing the little but noticeable changes for the better in the lives of the people I work with. By this, I mean that meeting their hearts with a gentle touch of kindness and a warm smile for reassurance makes all the difference. What I am saying is that I don't have to touch all the people, but if I can touch a person with my smile, then I have touched a million persons and empowered them to go and move another million persons just with the touch of a smile.

This attitude of mine makes the people I work with feel valued and appreciated because for some of them, my approach may be the first time in ages anyone has ever made them feel human in ages or met them with a genuine sense of empathy and left them with a heartfelt handshake or a hug to enforce that they are not alone. Mind you, I'll have to check if a hug or a handshake is what they need or if they just to be spoken to and heard. As a Christian, I bring solidarity and work with the mind of Christ.

You are currently writing a book titled _My Mental Health Matter: Beginnings_. Please tell us – what is this book about, why have you chosen to write it, and when can we expect it to be released?

My Mental Health Matter: Beginnings is a memorial of God's marvellous works in my life and in the lives of some of the people whom I am privileged to have met. This book, _Beginnings_, is about the beginning of God's revelation to me in a different dimension. In the pages, you will read about my period of healing and my journey into wholeness with Jesus Christ. So a part of this book consists of some elements of my relationship with Jesus Christ, and other aspects of it tell of some of my struggles in life, which are illustrated through poetry and testimonies of how I overcame physical health torments, as well as the impact on my mental health after I lost my elder brother to suicide in 2010.

For me, writing this book completes the remaining part of my healing process following the traumatic episodes I suffered after the loss of my late brother. After losing my elder brother, I suffered mental torture that tormented me into isolation and muteness.

The release date for this book was originally 2 October 2020, but the events that occurred during the course of this journey in the race to meet this date meant that this book in your hands today has been delivered to you now at the appointed time.

What advice do you have for women listening, especially those who might be going through depression?

Trust that the voice of the Most High will never lead you to destruction or tell you to take your life no matter the circumstances. I will say to never be shy to ask someone trusting to lend a hearing ear. However, before you run to any man or woman, there is a supernatural being who is indeed closer, the Holy Ghost. So my advice is to lean on and cry to God first; then trust God to direct you on how to resolve this issue and wait for His direction because He may sometimes use the simplest things to give you answers, and those things are mostly around you or within your reach, so obedience to God is paramount. I give a lot of nuggets and awareness on the topic of depression in the MentalHealthMatter. com blog.

Do you have any COVID-19 testimonies to share with people to encourage them to stay in the faith?

There are so many COVID-19 testimonies that I could share if I can remember them all. This is an indication that there are too many of them, but I would like to share this testimony about a time I visited the hospital and what led to it.

I was on my way back from a Sunday church service when I thought, 'I must go to the hospital to see how I can help.' I had been saying to myself that it would be a shame for me to go to the hospital for trivial matters when people in other nations are being rushed there in numbers because of serious life-threatening admissions from COVID-19.

I had this on my mind for a little while, but suddenly, prompting from the Holy Spirit came upon me, and the message it carried was a reminder not to go home until I had walked to a hospital to ask them how I could be of service during the pandemic. I did not want to disobey, so I did as I was reminded before going to visit my sibling.

When I walked into the hospital, I saw a woman I had known for years walking out of the hospital. She used to work at the post office counter but told me that she was now working at the hospital pharmacy. Upon my entrance to the hospital building, I was stopped, but after the course of my visit was established, I was directed to pick up some leaflets about volunteering with the chaplaincy team. The chaplaincy office was closed, but there was some information left out, so I picked one with a number on it and contacted this team. I was told that all volunteering with this team had been suspended because of the COVID-19 government restrictions, but they would keep me posted for future reopening and recruitment.

I left the hospital premises and told God that He is the supreme master over all and that I trust that He would make a way for me to volunteer in the NHS so that the pressure and workload on the shoulders of the staff would be reduced. My mind could not shift away from my visit to the hospital, so I called that number on the leaflet on Monday, 23 March 20. A reverend spoke with and gave me swift directions for the recruitment that would occur in an unforeseen date, so I waited.

To my greatest surprise, on 24 March 2020, I heard the news that Boris Johnson was seeking people to volunteer in the NHS sector to help bring the mania to a calm. This aired on 25 March 2020 on BBC News Online, titled 'Coronavirus Pandemic': 'Speaking at his daily news conference, PM Boris Johnson said all 504,303 could now play an "absolutely crucial" role . . . Mr Johnson said he wanted to offer [a] "special thank-you to everyone who has now volunteered to help the HNS".' I began to dance like a kid around my room. I thanked God for the quick answer to my prayers and for using the Holy Spirit to push me into obedience.

Fast-forwarding this testimony, God saw in my heart that I do pray for the sick to get up, make their beds, walk out of the hospital, and walk into their destinies and purposes for life. In conclusion, my faith carries a big section in this book, and I have carried my readers all the way throughout this book, letting them know how this is the most important aspect of my being because it has led to my wholeness and the birth of my ministry.

Thank you for talking with us, Merisha. How can the readers contact you to find out more about your work?

MyMentalHealthMatter.com

◐ Last Page ◉

Zachariah 4:10 in the New Living Translation Bible tells us what God says we should not do when we begin: 'Do not despite those small beginnings, for the Lord rejoices to see the work begin, to see the plumb line [in] Zerubbabl's hand.'

Change your disposion so that your position can change. I am glad I began this book. I am glad that God kept me on it. I am glad that I finished it. You start, and God will aid you to bring it to completion with the speed of the Holy Ghost.

'Whatever He asks you to do, just do it.'

—John 2:5 (paraphrased)

◐ At Last ◉

Congratulations for picking up this book and reading it until the last page!

I congratulate you for being alive. Know that you are worthy on earth and that heaven will remember and reward you.

I congratulate you for giving your life to Christ. If you have not already done so, I welcome you to do so using the simple prayer at the beginning of this book.

I offer you congratulations now that you are safe in Christ. When you move, God moves, just like that. Nobody gets a prize for knowing. It is through demonstrating what you know that the prize is won. **Be a winner.**

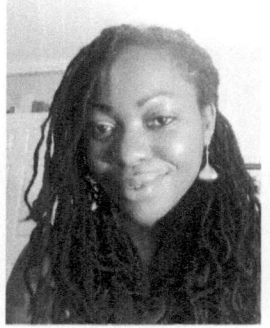

About the Author

Merisha Meisha

Bachelor of Acts in Creative Industries

Diploma in Theraputic Arts (Child and Adult)

Diploma in Health and Social Care (Child and Adult)

Competent Phlebotomist

Diploma Leadership in the Bible/Word of Faith

 This book forms part of the First People
Mental Health Wellness blog.

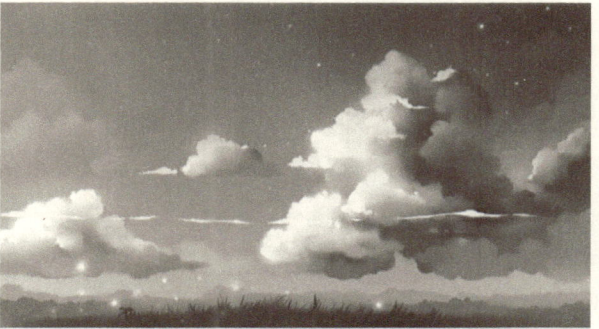

About the Book

Beginnings

This book, **_Beginnings_**, is a testimonial of God and His marvellous works in my life.

This book forms part of the First People Mental Health Wellness blog and People's People Ministires.

Word Translation Page

Pidgin English Translations

Oga — A senior man (used to show respect when addressing a person of authority).

Haba! — Come on!

Index

G

Galilee 9

Gath 34

God ix, xi, xiv-xvii, xix, xxi-xxiii, xxvii-xxxiii, xxxv-2, 4-20, 22-34, 36-85, 87-91, 93-6, 98-113, 115-36, 138-46, 149-51, 158, 160-71, 174-5, 180-1, 183-4, 188, 191, 205-20, 222-43, 246, 248-9, 251-3, 257-9, 261-71, 274, 279, 283-4, 286-8, 292-5, 299

Greenwich 12, 153, 172

Greenwich Home Start 288

H

Hammersmith 215

Holy Spirit xxxix, 5-7, 11, 14-15, 18-20, 23-5, 27-9, 31, 36-7, 39-41, 44, 46, 51, 54-5, 59, 72, 75, 82, 88, 115, 126, 129, 134, 160-1, 163-4, 168, 210, 213, 217-18, 227, 234-6, 240, 242, 244-5, 248, 252, 255, 258-9, 261, 263, 265, 269, 271, 291, 293-4

Human Genome Project 171

J

Jesus xv, xvii, 107, 124, 126, 128, 130, 133, 165, 169, 171, 181, 184, 205-6, 209-12, 215, 217, 220, 224-5, 227-30, 236, 248, 252-5, 262, 264, 276, 288, 292

K

Kent xxi, 13, 206, 208, 229-30

L

Lagos State 35, 146, 153-5

Lekki Beach 146, 149, 153

Lekki massacre 146, 149, 151, 153

Living Faith Bible Church xxi

London xv, xvii, xix, 12, 145, 147, 158, 161, 163, 172, 206, 208-9, 212, 216, 218-19, 221-3, 226, 230, 271, 281-2

M

Metro Bank 161

My Mental Health Matter xxvi, 119, 287

N

New Cross Railway Station xix

New Jerusalem 90

Nigeria 12, 35, 145-7, 153, 155-6, 158, 183, 228, 268

O

Orpington 206

P

Pen to Print 282

People's People Mind Gap xiv

Princess Royal university hospital 206

Q

queen elizabeth hospital 212, 214-15

Queen's Hospital 226

R

Romford 226

Royal Borough Greenwich London 271

Royal Mail 265

Royal Woolwich Arsenal Station 218

S

Siloam 22

Sweden xvii-xviii, xxv, 208

T

Tottenham Spurs   221

U

United Kingdom   xix, xxv, 146-7, 268

W

WHSmith   244

Winners Chapel   xvi, xxi, 12, 207-8, 215, 291

Woolwich   214, 218, 222, 229

www.ingramcontent.com/pod-product-compliance
Lightning Source LLC
Chambersburg PA
CBHW021349210526
45463CB00001B/35